GREAT BODY FOR SENIORS

Develop Your Best Body and Health Over 65

LOYALTY: giving or showing firm and constant support or allegiance to a person
"He remained loyal to her for 34 years"

Chris R. Rea

ReaShape

Copyright © Chris Rea 2014.

All rights reserved. No part of this book may be used or reproduced in any manner whatsoever without written permission.

ISBN: 978-0-9903094-2-0

The nutritional and health information in this book is based on the author's experiences. It is intended only as a guide and is not meant to replace the advice of a physician, dietitian, physical therapist, or other health professional. Always seek competent professional help if you have concerns about the appropriateness of this information for you.

Printed in the United States of America

Dedication

To my mother.

Contents

Introduction	7
1. Quality of Life: Our Ultimate Goal	9
2. A Committed Lifestyle	14
3. How Can We Become Motivated?	23
4. Reprogramming the Mind	28
5. Developing the Game Plan	34
6. The Diet	41
7. Different Diets for Different People	55
8. The Difference between Men and Women	71
9. Feeling the Difference	80
10. Meal Frequency and Portions	89
11. Carbohydrates and Fast Weight Loss	95
12. Sculpting Your Body	126
13. Calisthenics Training	165
14. Supersetting	179
15. Putting It All Together	202
16. Reaping the Benefits	207

Introduction

Individuals have two contrasting thoughts when they hear the term "aging". The first thought of aging is at the positive end of the spectrum-experience and wisdom comes with age. Because experience and wisdom positively and beneficially correlate with age, we learn more about ourselves, in particular, and more about life, in general. The second thought of aging is the the negative end of the spectrum. Individuals tend to associate again with the loss of knowledge, confidence, and experience rather than the attainment of them. More specifically, the negative thoughts on aging focus on the loss of our physical strength and faculties as well as problems related to our mental cognition and consciousness, such as memory loss and declining cognitive function.

The truth is that is that society perceives aging more as a sadness of loss than a happiness of benefit.

The association of older age as being the years in decline does not have to be the case at all. We have the ability to slow down the aging process by making some adaptations to our lifestyle to make it different—and better. To achieve a different lifestyle means making a few changes, both physically and mentally. Changing your lifestyle by making physical changes has an immediate impact on the way you feel. As you begin to feel physically much better due to the new lifestyle changes, you then feel the mental changes simultaneously. These physical and mental changes will begin to transform your life by improving your quality of life.

The term "quality of life" has enormous depth and value in its meaning. We all want to feel and look better because this will improve our sense of well-being and confidence, which in turn makes us feel happier overall. Have you ever heard the saying, "Happiness can bring you wealth but wealth will never bring you happiness?" It's true. Happiness is the foundation for a solid structure in life. Happiness isn't something we are born with, but rather, it's the result of an accumulation of positive effort, positive behavior, and a healthy lifestyle. Living a healthy lifestyle is what I am about to teach you. It's what this book is all about, because a healthy lifestyle leads to our ultimate goal, maintaining a good quality of life as we age.

Chapter 1
Quality of Life: Our Ultimate Goal

The term quality of life carries a lot of meaning and value to me now. It didn't always. When I was growing up, my father would talk about quality of life often. He would say that this was our goal and what we were striving for, but never did it resonate with me, a typical American kid. My father had a different mindset. As an immigrant from Spain, with its beautiful culture, my father had grown up in a part of the world where quality of life, not wealth or possessions, was the ultimate goal.

To my father, quality of life meant the overall happiness that comes from the way they live. What makes their life have such pleasure and value is the happiness and enjoyment factor. Western Europeans are world-renowned for the way they live. To be more specific, European traditions put an emphasis on quality as opposed to quantity.

Americans often aspire to the luxuries that make our lives more comfortable. We want a comfortable home, nice clothing, and good food. If they have those, most people consider they have a good quality of life. My interpretation, however, is slightly different from the norm, because I place a much larger importance on health and fitness. I certainly agree that a comfortable home, nice clothing, and good food do indeed play key roles in having a high standard of living. I would definitely include exercise and proper nutrition into that same formula. Proper nutrition and exercise combined equal a winning combination.

Eating Well
Let's begin with nutrition. When we think of good food, we imag-

ine exotic five-star dishes we would eat in the best restaurants. Many people would also think of good food as being home-cooked—we all love Mom's cooking. But is good food always nutritious food? Often good refers to the taste rather than the nutritional value. I don't mean nutritious food tastes bad; what I mean is that good food isn't always good for you. Foods that taste very good are usually high in calories and lower in nutritional value, while foods that are low in calories and high in nutritional value tend not to be as tasty.

How does nutrition play an important part in having a good quality of life as we get older? In several ways, starting with having improved health, which should be our main priority. Without health our lives are much more limited or even worse, and can come to an abrupt ending. The difference between poor and good health is substantial, and the difference between good and great health is also enormous.

To be more specific, someone in good health may function well but feel mediocre throughout the day. Someone who is in exceptional health will thrive throughout the same day, instead of just survive. Being in great shape gives you ample energy and strength to really get the most out of the typical day. Instead of just making it through the day, someone in good condition has many more options, such as playing sports, walking, and other high-energy and youthful activities. Eating properly will instantly provide more energy and confidence throughout your day.

Exercise is another extremely important element for having a good quality of life. Regular exercise will provide increased energy and a decreased chance of bodily injury. With exercise, the body gets stronger and better coordinated. That strengthens you and prevents injuries and falls. As we age, injuries need to be avoided at all costs. Having a fit and strong body will let you continue with or even begin activities you used to only dream of doing.

Proper nutrition and exercise are crucial elements for improving your life. When you get a nutritionally balanced diet and have a proper exercise routine, within a surprisingly short time your body will feel as if it has just discovered the fountain of youth. Let's admit it, feeling and looking young is an important element in your quality of life. As you age, it's great to keep the energy you had when you were younger.

Have you ever heard the saying, "Youth is wasted on the young?" How about when you were younger, and older people would say, "If I only knew then what I know now?" I used to hear that a lot when I was a young man. When I got a bit older, I realized that wishing I was younger and regretting the opportunities I had missed or not taken advantage of is part of maturing. I realized that yes, life can be quite sad, especially if we fall short of reaching our dreams and goals. But I also saw that many people didn't achieve their goals because they had health problems caused by poor diet and poor lifestyle. I realized that you can still have a positive, youthful attitude at any age. As people get older, they tend to overthink many situations, which makes them too cautious or too fearful of failure. These negative feelings can make older people stop pursuing their dreams and begin to feel they are simply too old for achieving new goals. An accumulation of such goal-preventing feelings eventually causes more sadness and possibly depression.

This sort of defeated feeling doesn't have to happen. Simply by altering your lifestyle and way of thinking, you make positive changes in your mindset and way of thinking. This can enable you to become a completely different person--a person with a positive attitude, enormous energy, and a winner's mentality that never quits! All of a sudden you feel young again. You now have that second chance at youth you always wanted. You can now do the things you regretted not doing when you were younger. You can do things you used to enjoy but haven't done recently because you thought that you were just too old. For you, age is now just a number, not how you feel. Wouldn't you want to have more freedom? The freedom to do more things, engage in more activities, and not have to rely on so many pills and medication? You can regain the freedom of youth and get moving in the morning without needing an hour to stretch out the aches and pains and another hour to take your meds and get dressed.

Freedom is a meaningful word and we seem to become less free as we age. If you're not in good condition as you age, you lose a lot of your freedom through limits on your activities, what you can eat, your energy levels, even the clothing you can wear comfortably. It doesn't have to be that way.

Health Equals Freedom

Whenever people think of freedom they imagine themselves having more time to do the things that they enjoy doing. This is true, but let's be a little more specific about what freedom means. Let's get to the core of freedom. What is necessary for us to have the ability to do the things we want? First and foremost, it's good health. This is where all opportunities begin. Of course, having financial freedom is important as well, but my answer to that is again, good health. When you are healthy, all goals seem possible. You can provide yourself with financial security because being healthy will allow you to work, preferably at the career of your choice, for as long and as hard as you want. You'll be able to keep working at the peak of your earning power, without having to cut back or retire early because of poor health or disability.

Achieving optimum physical health so you can stay active, whether that means continuing to work or retiring to enjoy your later years, includes proper nutrition and exercise. Let's start with a short summary about nutrition. The food you eat is equal to the fuel that powers a car. For example, a race car uses high-quality fuel to perform at the highest level. The same applies to the body. Compare eating a bag of potato chips to a eating a baked sweet potato. Both are made from healthy root vegetables, but the potato chips have had their nutrition processed away. They're filled with unwanted ingredients such as salt, sugar, processed oils, and preservatives that may harm the body. The unwanted ingredients in the chips are digested properly in the body, taking away from its performance. Think of using low-quality fuel in a race car; it will not run properly or at its full potential—the poor fuel might even damage the engine.

On the other end of the spectrum, your body will immediately notice the difference if you eat the sweet potato completely by itself, without additives. The sweet potato will be efficiently digested and provide the body with a steady flow of optimum nutrition and energy, just like using high-octane racing fuel in a racing car. Your body is designed for high-quality fuel, just as the race car is.

Simply by eating a healthier diet, you are about to open the door to an entirely new life, one with more energy, confidence, and a better appearance. If you add exercise to your healthy eating habits, the results will be amazing. On a daily basis you'll feel physical and emotional improvements that can last a lifetime. Whoever said growing old had to be a negative experience? This doesn't have to be the case at all. Rather than growing old, you can be "growing young." Of course, the process of growing young isn't going to happen overnight, nor will be easy. In order to age while staying as healthy as possible, and to reach the point where your body is actually improving to unprecedented levels, takes commitment and sacrifice. The payoff is more than worth it. Could you ever imagine waking up every morning with no pains, feeling fully energized, appearing and feeling years younger, and overall being happier? This is all possible. It's no secret. What prevents everyone from taking the path of rejuvenation is a fear of commitment and failure. Sadly, many older people lack confidence and no longer believe, if they ever did, that good health and high energy are still possible. Of course they are, but only if you are truly committed to improving how you feel.

Chapter 2
A Committed Lifestyle

Many people wish they could look and feel better but believe it is no longer possible when you become older. In reality, people are not satisfied with their appearance and the way they feel because the price they would need to pay for improvement would simply be too much. What is meant by price is commitment, sacrifice, and discipline. These three words tend to scare older people away.

At this point I'm sure you're thinking, why do I keep mentioning words such as "commitment" and "discipline"? You're reading this book simply as a means of getting into shape, losing weight, and feeling better. You would be expecting only to read about exercise routines and healthy diets. You do need a healthy diet and good exercise routines, but here's where I differ from any others in terms of how to approach getting into shape. I believe your approach begins from the "inside out," rather than simply the "outside." More specifically, my approach begins with the mind and way of thinking. This includes almost reprogramming your mind in a way that will help you positively affect everyday decisions and making adjusting to your new and healthier life seem as effortless as possible. "Growing young" and getting into phenomenal shape is not by any means an overnight process. It's a longer and gradual lifestyle adjustment. Perhaps these are not the words you would prefer to hear. Maybe you'd rather hear how my program is "fast," "easy," and "effortless." Unfortunately those appealing words are not the words of success. They're the words of short-term results followed by long-term disappointment and failure. Being in the best shape of your life requires quite a bit of commitment. Those who are willing to fully commit are the only people that I prefer to guide. My biggest thrill is guiding people toward achieving the best shape of their lives. Positive results are what motivate me.

Slow, Steady Progress

Results are necessary in order to achieve the ultimate goal, which is happiness. Quality of life is included with happiness and being healthy will get you there. My methods of achieving quality of life—happiness, looking better, feeling younger and healthier, and increasing overall confidence—are all part of the package that I am putting together for you. This package is a revolving door, because the elements all work together. Not one can be achieved without the other. Feeling fantastic, looking better than ever, and overall improving your life are all tied together.

We need to begin at the base, the core which is living a disciplined life of rigorous changes in diet and exercise. We must be clear on this, because you must be willing to commit. You must want to look and feel better in a big way. Living a life of sacrifice, discipline, and humility is necessary to improve your body and health to new levels, levels you never thought were possible to achieve even in your 20s and 30s. This may not seem possible—and it isn't unless you are fully committed, both mentally and physically. Success will not happen overnight. However, when it does occur, you will feel a transition, as though you have just awakened to a new and better life.

Every person has different goals they aspire to achieve. One goal isn't better than the next, because each individual has a different way of thinking.

Turning Back the Clock

How many times have we heard people say, "I wish that I could go back in time and re-live my youth." It's fun to reminisce about the good old days and how much better everything used to be. Well, why daydream about the past when these dreams can come true now, in the present and near future? Living a life filled with unachieved goals is what many people end up doing. That's what we definitely want to avoid. Having dreams and aspirations in life is what gives our life purpose, and with purpose comes drive and passion. We all have regrets. When asked what their biggest regret was, most people don't mention their failures in life. Instead, they say their biggest regrets were "the chances they never even took." This simple act of not even trying to accomplish a dream, or trying and failing, causes emotional regression.

When your dreams escape you time and time again, year after year, your emotional state begins to suffer and emotional regression occurs. With time, lack of confidence begins to hinder your happiness and zest. You start to look and feel defeated. Have you ever watched a sporting event and noticed at the end of the game how differently the winning and losing teams walk off the field? The winning team walks off the field with the swagger of confidence and a smile, while the defeated team walks off with their heads down, walking hunched over and with a frown. The winning team exudes a positive energy that attracts people, while the defeated team exudes a negative, energy-sapping force that people want to avoid.

Use this same formula with regular, everyday people. Ever notice how people always seem to be attracted and drawn to those who are goal-driven and accomplished while on the other hand, everyone seems to avoid those who frequently complain and have a tendency to either quit or lose? People always want to feel happy and energized, so they are drawn to those who exude positive energy and will avoid those who exude negative energy. Each dream begins with positive thinking and experiences. When people daydream they often think of their happiest moments and most successful accomplishments. Who enjoys daydreaming of unhappy moments? It does make sense to think about negative experiences in order to learn from your mistakes and avoid repeating them. But it's more useful and more enjoyable to daydream and reminisce about best past moments and future aspirations. Daydreaming is necessary for growth. When we spend time thinking about both our past experiences and future goals, we enable ourselves to set higher goals and plan ways to make them a reality. Without dreams and ideas, we won't progress much, thus living a life of simple routine and without excitement.

How does all this pertain to health and fitness? Happiness and quality of life will result from optimum physical and mental health and a proper exercise program. Combining them all makes the winning mix of happiness, productivity, and looking and feeling great.

The Importance of Structure

Having solid structure in your life is the equivalent of a house having a solid foundation. What happens when a house isn't built on a solid foundation? Eventually, it begins to fall apart. The same applies to structure and the human body. A solid structure for the body means having adequate sleep, proper nutrition, and sufficient exercise. These three parts combined together create a strong foundation for the body which then leads to having a more productive and happier life, which, in turn, means an improved quality of life. You'll be amazed what a difference having a solid foundation and structure will make. Once you start sleeping, eating, and exercising regularly, you realize how much everything else in your life improves. Once you start feeling the benefits of these improvements, you'll want more. You'll want to learn how to eat an even healthier diet, exercise more intensely, and sleep more soundly.

When all three elements are combined, the body suddenly begins to operate more efficiently. The word "efficient" is the exact opposite of the word "waste," because waste is something we always want to avoid. Any type of waste, whether of time, energy, money, or anything else, will lead to inefficiency, unhappiness, and frustration.

Simply stated, we want to avoid waste while we implement efficiency. We always want to improve. I have never heard of a business shutting its doors because it was running too efficiently, but there have been many that have gone out of business because there was too much waste.

Creating Structure

Creating proper structure is the foundation for any type of success. The real secret is to create a structure that works for *you*. For example, people often explain and recommend their daily structure of exercise, sleep, and nutrition to me because it is what made *them* achieve their goals and success. I do appreciate the gesture and it is very uplifting to know people want to help me. I often get good tips from them, but these people usually have completely different goals, tastes, and schedules as compared to mine. Their structure works for them, but it's not conducive for me to follow.

To create the structure that works best for you, you will have to go through some time-consuming trial-and-error. If you pay attention to what works and what doesn't, this trial-and-error phase won't be too long. My process took years only because my knowledge was acquired by reading many books, several years of competitive college wrestling, body building competitions, and mixed martial arts competitions. This long process was truly beneficial because I acquired knowledge from many different sports, from different countries, and from different experts in their field. For me, this trial-and-error phase eventually transformed into seeking perfection phase, because I have always been extremely interested in gaining ever more knowledge. Teaching and helping people achieving optimum health is my biggest passion.

In this book, I have narrowed down all my years of experience achieving optimum health into a "fast track" system. Each year, it becomes easier for me to achieve great physical health, thanks to all the prior years of trial and error I endured.

In fitness as in everything else, we look to find the quicker and easier way. There are no shortcuts toward achieving your goals, but there are more efficient ways. Over the years, I've found efficient ways that help shorten the process while making it easier at the same time. My program not only works, it's "user-friendly." I have effectively concentrated this formula by combining only the diet and exercise programs that work best.

Sleep, Food, Exercise

Creating the proper structure is where we began. Think of three main words: sleep, food, exercise.

Sleeping is an important investment in your health. During sleep, the body repairs itself and releases all of the necessary hormones that are needed for the body to operate at its best. Sleeping seven to eight hours every night will render tremendous health benefits. During sleep, the brain dreams as a way to discharge the stress of the day. Your brain also clears out metabolic waste products while you sleep—think of it as taking out the brain's trash. The body releases a growth hormone responsible for rejuvenation while you sleep. Growth hormones provide the skin with the elasticity we tend to lose as we age. Wouldn't you want to have firm, tight skin again? You can definitely make a difference by sleeping enough.

Hormones, chemical messengers in your body, are also responsible for burning body fat and for developing muscle mass. Both of these functions by themselves should have you interested, because losing body fat and gaining muscle is our goal. Maximizing the body's hormones is the hidden secret to achieving great health, fitness, and quality of life. To do this, sleeping and waking at the same time every day, like clockwork, is a must.

So, phase one is making the decision to create structure and get into shape. The second phase is sleeping seven to eight hours per night, always at the same time, in order for your body to create the perfect circadian (day/night) rhythm.

Creating a healthy routine and circadian rhythm is very important for the body. This will enable you to bring your body to its peak potential. Regardless of the time of day you sleep, eat, and exercise, it is important to maintain exactly the same schedule each day. Create a steady and constant routine. Going to sleep and awaking at the same time daily is the first step toward creating a healthy structure. Think of sleeping as an investment, because the time you spend asleep will make the remaining hours of the day much more effective. It will lead to increased efficiency, more energy, a happier mood, more patience, and a much healthier appearance.

For men, sleeping adequately also increases the body's natural production of testosterone which is the male hormone linked to an increased libido, strength, mood, and energy. When the body's natural hormones are at peak levels, the body will feel and perform years younger. Have you ever wondered why someone in his twenties seems to be strong, energetic, and have a positive outlook, while a much older person seems to be weaker in strength, energy and have a less happy personality? This change occurs mainly because of the body's decreasing levels of testosterone and growth hormone production. This does not have to be the case at all, because by taking care of the body you can naturally increase its hormone production. More hormones mean the body responds by feeling stronger, happier, healthier, and younger.

Does this sound too good to be true? Perhaps, but I'm not a snake oil salesman. I'm not saying this will happen overnight or without effort. To improve your body and mood, you will have to commit, make sacrifices, and expect to maintain a very disciplined life. To reverse the aging process, you must be willing to be dedicated.

Here's what occurs when the body doesn't receive adequate sleep: natural testosterone and human growth hormone production is decreased, facial skin will not have a healthy glow, you will become less patient, more depressed, and more tired—and less productive. Think of spiraling down toward a crash landing. Not sleeping enough, particularly deep REM (rapid eye movement) sleep doesn't allow the brain to dream enough. You can't unload and reprogram your brain, which then causes decreased cognitive function. Your memory will decrease, and you will have less ability to effectively concentrate, add numbers rapidly, and many other side effects of decreased cognitive function.

Without adequate sleep, the body releases more of a hormone called cortisol. Often called the stress hormone, cortisol is the hormone that triggers the "fight or flight" mode. In short bursts, cortisol is normal and necessary—it's what lets you respond quickly in an emergency, for example. But when you're under constant stress and don't get enough sleep, your cortisol levels go up and stay up. That causes the nervous system to overreact. That in turn makes your body's metabolism shift away from maintaining and building muscle and toward storing fat. When cortisol levels are high, you have less patience, you become extremely sleepy during the afternoon, your memory and ability to study or perform difficult mental tasks is tremendously hindered. If I don't get enough sleep because of stress, my workouts at the gym are sluggish. I don't feel the pump, the sign that lactic acid is building up in my muscles because they're getting a good workout. I become very depressed. All of a sudden, I look at life as a gloomy experience, I have no drive to do anything and just get through the day by going through the motions, without any zest or passion. I end up being very unproductive that day, which only adds to the depression that I was already feeling. But if that night I sleep seven to eight restful hours, I wake up feeling like a completely new and better person, with a much better outlook and way of thinking. It's as if my firepower just magically came back!

The reason a good night's sleep is the first step toward getting into phenomenal shape and spirit is because, not only is sleeping the easiest and most fun (providing you had a fun dream especially) part of the process, without enough sleep nothing else will work. You won't be able to get to the next step in the quest to feel and look better and younger.

Motivation Fuels Success

Sleep is an extremely important investment, because without adequate sleep it will become nearly impossible to reach your goals. Whenever I don't sleep enough it negatively affects my mood and this alone is a tremendous disadvantage. Without enough sleep, I become much less patient. Wherever I may be at that particular moment, I am not comfortable at all. Instead, I'm waiting for new stimulation, eager to get to the next place instead of paying attention to where I am. What ends up happening is my day is wasted. For example, if my day is filled with meetings and exercise along with social events, if I'm at a meeting and have to go to the gym to exercise, as soon as the meeting ends, my mind isn't on reviewing the decisions; instead, I'm thinking that I can't wait to get to the gym. At the gym, my workouts are subpar at best. I'm only going through the motions because I'm already eager to finish to go eat lunch. At lunch, I don't enjoy the meal because my mind is already thinking about the meeting I have to go to following lunch. At the meeting, I'm already eager to leave to go on to the next place.

Because I didn't sleep enough, wherever I am is not where I want to be; my patience becomes nonexistent. What really occurs is my day is wasted, my quality of life is poor, and I become more depressed because the day was not productive at all for me and the people I was with. Now multiply this by ten years of not enough sleep. You've pretty much wasted ten years because your body wasn't functioning 100 percent. Unfortunately, this happens to many people every day simply because they aren't sleeping enough. Without adequate sleep, you are only surviving, not thriving, but is only thriving that brings happiness, success, and quality of life. Surviving brings only the minimum needed for you to barely function in a life laden with responsibilities. Sufficient sleep increases energy and mood, which combined together, increase motivation. Passion combined with motivation enables you to reach new levels of happiness, success, and quality of life.

Chapter 3
How Can We Become Motivated?

Motivation is a key element needed for both success and quality of life. Success is achieved through performance, and peak performance is achieved through both passion and motivation. When people are motivated they tend to excel in what they are motivated in, because whatever motivates them they have passion for. This circular effect will become easier to understand as I explain the process of achieving success (which brings happiness and improves quality of life) from both the beginning to the top, and from the success right down to the very beginning of the process.

Let's start from the very beginning. This begins with an idea, a dream, an aspiration. Simply thinking of this already puts you into a good mood and perhaps even gives you a smile. discipline, and sacrifice. Here is where most people fail before they really start, because they aren't willing to commit themselves to working toward their dream and they don't feel confident enough in themselves to remain committed. The unfortunate truth is most people don't have the necessary confidence to believe that they can achieve their goals simply because they fear the commitment that is required.

When we watch a professional athlete, performer, or movie star, we tend to think this famous person became successful simply by good luck or that they were special or "gifted" individuals. We think their attainments are out of the question for us. Thinking this way will automatically shatter your hopes of achieving any of your dreams and goals. The famous people you admire achieved success through endless hours of hard work and many failures and setbacks along the way. They succeeded because they had a dream and a plan to reach that dream without ever quitting. Each of these people had passion for that dream. They were highly motivated to spend the necessary time and energy required to succeed, and they did it for the love and the passion. Financial reward wasn't their primary motivation. In fact, many passed up other opportunities so they could pursue their dream. What was their motivation? Their passion.

Always remember that having strong motivation is required to feel and perform at peak levels. Motivation is the driving force for happiness and success. But what makes people become powerfully motivated? They choose to do what they enjoy most. Of course, we must also be realistic about what we enjoy doing, otherwise everyone would choose an enjoyable activity such as going on vacation as their career. You won't make progress that way. Making your own decisions based on your own choice of the best possible options will slowly guide you into a lifestyle that is most comfortable for you. That will enable you to become more motivated to live a more productive life, which in turn will enable you to achieve more and increase your happiness and quality of life.

Being motivated simply enables you to get more out of the 24 hours in each and every day. Motivation will increase your confidence and confidence increases your quality of life. Motivation, passion, commitment, discipline, and hard work, when combined together, lead to a much better life.

What motivates me is my passion for helping you achieve optimum health and fitness so you can have your best-looking, best-feeling body ever, regardless of your age. It's never too late. If you have the will, the drive, and the passion, I will show you the way!

Passion

To become successful and happier, you need passion, because passion creates motivation. It's very difficult to succeed in things that we don't have passion for. Regardless of your goals and activities, there is always a way to find passion and motivation. It may become difficult to find passion in activities you have no interest in, but with creativity you can always find a way. For example, my passion is the best health and fitness, so being in shape is an important part of my life. Overall, I enjoy the process because getting into and maintaining great health is something I care about, but there are things about the process I don't enjoy. When I don't enjoy something, I can always find a way to alter the part that isn't that much fun. I look for ways to vary the routine in ways that are better and easier for me. Let's say, for instance, that I need to do cardio every day in order to achieve my ultimate passion of being in shape, but the most common means of cardio training, such as running on a treadmill, really bore me. How can I make cardio more fun? Simple: By finding a cardiovascular exercise that's enjoyable for me, such as riding a bicycle.

Another example would be my diet. Let's just say that I don't enjoy eating egg whites for breakfast, but I do need to eat some type of protein for breakfast. So what should I do? The egg whites can be switched to whey protein powder as my new source of protein for breakfast.

A few simple and creative changes can create or reignite a passion. Switching to riding a bicycle and having a protein shake made me look forward to having Breakfast and doing my cardio. With this change I now have more passion and am more motivated to get into even better shape.

To have passion, you need to be deeply interested in a particular hobby, activity, or goal. My passion is health and fitness. All of us have a talent or passion we can choose to excel in. Even if you're not passionate about or interested in health and fitness, I'm willing to bet that you have a strong interest in looking and feeling your very best. Admit it, you want to have a leaner body and be more attractive. But if none of your passions and interests lie in health and fitness, we have to get creative to motivate you to exercise and diet. This includes choosing the healthy foods that are tastiest to you and the exercises that are most fun for you to perform. People often aren't successful with a diet and exercise program because they follow one that was recommended for them, rather than one that was custom-made for them. You will be far more successful following a program that's fun, not boring.

You've probably heard the expression "no pain, no gain" when it comes to getting into shape. To a degree, this is true. Yes, you will need to make sacrifices to improve your body and health, but the secret is to carefully choose the right options that will make these sacrifices easier. This is why being creative when constructing a meal plan and workout routine is very important for achieving success.

Creativity and Passion

To succeed you must love what you do. To become good at anything you need motivation and passion. Just about everyone wants to have a nicer and healthier body, but if that is the only thing they want, then the quest will become nearly impossible to achieve. To create a lean and healthy physique, you must have discipline and patience because this is required for the entire process. Don't expect to lose body fat and tone your body unless commitment is involved.

Start by reprogramming the negative feelings inside your mind. You must envision yourself already having the body and health you have always wanted. Everything begins in the mind with positive thinking. Prior to even beginning a workout and food regimen, you must envision yourself having a fantastic body and health. What this does is develop and reprogram your subconscious mind. To give an analogy of the mind's machinations, think of a river with a powerful undertow. This river may seem calm on the surface, but once you attempt to swim it, a force rapidly drags you downstream with a current too great to swim against. The subconscious works the same way. On the outside you may believe you want to lose weight and get into shape, but your subconscious doesn't allow you to. It prefers that you do what has always been easiest, such as being lazy and not committed.

Your self-esteem is also connected to your subconscious, which makes you lack the confidence needed to succeed. Therefore, rather than risk failure, your mind prevents you from engaging in such tasks.

Years upon years of taking the easy way out has programmed your mind in a negative way. In order to succeed, we must first reprogram your mind so it will motivate your subconscious in a positive way. Every type of success begins at ground zero, your mind.

Chapter 4
Reprogramming the Mind

Before beginning the journey to a lifestyle of health and fitness, you must first believe in yourself. Confidence is necessary and, as progress occurs, your confidence increases. To reprogram the mind, only positive thoughts and successful visualization should occupy much of your thinking. You must "believe in order to achieve." If your mind is not reprogrammed in a positive way, then your exercise and nutritional program will be short-lived. More than likely you will give up and stop dieting and exercising seriously as soon as you feel the slightest pain or mental challenge. In the world of health and fitness, results don't come overnight.

Mind reprogramming consists of positive and patient thinking; this will increase your confidence. Thinking positively and confidently will make you believe in yourself and feel that completing any task or goal is within your reach. Confidence is acquired by successfully completing tasks, from small to large. It's good practice to work toward completing goals and tasks on a constant basis. Begin by completing small tasks. Setting small and reachable goals such as cleaning your room, organizing the closet, paying the bills on time, having the car serviced, losing one pound per week, saving one dollar per week, and doing any other small task that can be completed in a short amount of time.

What happens when you do this is that, without even realizing it, your confidence is increasing, because you're accomplishing all the small tasks and goals that you've set for yourself. By completing ordinary daily tasks, are you becoming more responsible and your confidence is also increasing. You're mentally preparing yourself for the successful journey of getting into phenomenal shape. Your mind is reprogramming itself, transforming you into a confident warrior who is now ready for successful battle—the creation of an unbelievable body and health.

Stagnation Halts Success
What we want to avoid during this process is any type of stagnation, or lack of movement and growth. Humans are happiest when they have meaningful work and are productive, which is the opposite of stagnation. Sadly, many people are products of stagnation simply because there has been no steady and constant growth in their lives. At all costs, we must work toward progress, otherwise the opposite occurs--regression and stagnation. When we are moving forward and progressing, we feel happy and accomplished. Why wouldn't you want to feel this way constantly? Because negative thoughts of failure and lack of confidence enter the mind and cause laziness. This is a feeling we must avoid at all costs. Confidence defeats laziness every time.

Think of a salesperson and failure. A salesperson must accept rejection and failure constantly, without ever losing hope and always feeling sure that the sales will come in the end. Even the best salespeople experience rejection much more often than making a sale, but they accept this and continue on the path toward success. Failure is a part of success. In fact, you can learn and improve a lot more from failure than from success.

Don't let the fear of failure create a life of stagnation, because eventually stagnation causes depression. For example, ever notice how many people only speak about their children's accomplishments in school, sports or even physical growth, such as their height? The conversation is never about themselves, only the children? Partly this is because all parents love to brag about their kids, but it's also because the parents are living in stagnation and boredom. The only progression they can speak about is the growth of their children. Again, parents to this because they love their kids, but also because they enjoy being a part of progression and productivity. Rather than living vicariously through the children, why not live in progression in your own life as well?

Stagnation and Depression

Constantly working toward and making consistent progress makes us happier and more confident. What causes stagnation is a combination of lack of confidence and fear of failure. Regardless of the size of the task, it is important to consistently work toward improvement. We're only human, so we can't ever achieve perfection, but we can aim for constant improvement.

At this point you're probably wondering why you're reading this book. So far there's been nothing about losing weight and toning the body—no exercise routines and healthy food options. That's because I want you to create a solid and long-lasting foundation to your diet and workout regimen, one that will last you a lifetime and lessen your chances of failure. In other words, we are starting from the ground up! I have kept in shape and helped many others for most of my lifetime. I know that we need to design a program that works for you. We can't do that unless you have a strong foundation. That begins with your mind, how it works, and how to reprogram it to increase your drive, passion, motivation, discipline, and determination. If your mind is ready, it is all possible, regardless of age. Never doubt your abilities or use your age as an excuse to stop yourself from achieving the body that you always dreamed about.

If you're motivated you can accomplish anything, because motivation provides the needed drive. Motivation is the opposite of stagnation. You must continually seek improvement and progress in everyday life, otherwise you will begin to regress. Most people are either progressing or regressing in life. Rarely do they remain in a neutral state. Progression usually brings happiness, while regression brings depression. For your health and wellbeing, it is very important to be continually working toward progression. Stagnation must be avoided at all costs, because its side effects are a depressed mood and way of thinking.

If you are not progressing, then stagnation begins. Eventually you notice that your life is stalled. Then you begin to overthink the situation and have a lot of negativity. Once your mind is filled with negative thinking, such as "Why am I not improving?" or "Why am I sad?" you eventually begin to spiral into depression. Depression is a feeling that you want to avoid at all costs, because this is a quick way to drastically destroy your quality of life. A chain reaction occurs: when people are depressed, they look for ways to get their mind away from the sadness by escaping, often in harmful or unhealthy ways. Escaping sadness and depression becomes a part of everyday life. Unfortunately, these escapes are merely short-term solutions. Escaping usually makes the depression worse because during the escapes, people are usually unproductive. After the mental escape, you are right back to where you began.

Escapes can be productive, but often they are detrimental. Unfortunately, most people choose the escapes that tend to be "short-term gains but long-term pains." In other words, people choose to escape without being productive. Unproductive escapism causes stagnation, which then leads to depression. For example, when most people feel sad or stressed, they want to forget about the misery, rather than attack the problem and work toward fixing it. During difficult moments, this is why people often turn having few drinks in order to forget about everything. Alcohol is probably the most common means of escapism, but there are many more; often, those who are escaping aren't even aware of it. Other unproductive forms of escaping could be shopping excessively, gambling, excessive dating and socializing, frequent traveling, watching television, using the Internet, listening to music and any other activity that takes your mind away from reality. You trade a few moments of pleasure, but you don't make any substantial improvement in your life.

Those who choose alcohol or drugs (including the abuse of prescription medication) eventually realize that their problems only become worse. The moment the effects of the alcohol or drugs wear off, the person feels much worse. Use of these substances leads to even more depression. This is why alcohol, in particular, is classified as a depressant. Gambling would also be considered a detrimental addiction. The mind is occupied, but only temporarily and in an unproductive way. The drawbacks far outweigh the benefits. Another form of escape is compulsive shopping. Shoppers feel a sudden and short-lived rush and stimulation that momentarily takes the mind away from the everyday sadness and into the feeling of action and stimulation. This rush comes to a sudden end after the purchase and an even more sudden end as soon as the payment needs to be made.

Many people use excessive socializing as a form of escaping reality. They may go to a lot of social events, give a lot of parties to hold, talk endlessly on the phone, date constantly, taking too many weekend trips and vacations (I was guilty of this), spend hours web surfing and playing Internet games, and engage in a lot of other excessive social behavior that only leads to daily stagnation.

All types and forms of escaping reality have two things in common: They all provide a quick burst of temporary happiness, and they enable you to hide from responsibilities. Think of an alcoholic or a drug addict needing that quick fix to satisfy the urge. The same applies to stimulation junkies, who are constantly looking for an escape. The quick fix, the instant gratification, and stimulation is exactly what we need to avoid. By doing this, we are running further away from completing hard-earned goals and accomplishments that could lead us to happiness. Focus on working on long-term goals and accomplishments. Instant gratification leads to a lifetime of never reaching your true potential; instead, you can end up spending a lifetime chasing one quick rush of instant gratification after the other. Next thing you realize, your life is almost over and your goals and dreams were never achieved. Throughout this entire process you can never become truly happy, but instead keep falling deeper into living a subpar life.

On the other end of the spectrum, if you imagine a goal and carefully plan how it will be achieved, then carefully work toward completing that goal, you begin to enjoy the entire journey. As each small improvement is noticed and each step is completed, that leads to more confidence and happiness every step of the way. The continual process of seeking achievement slowly creates a solid foundation that eventually leads to true and everlasting success, happiness, and quality of life!

Chapter 5
Developing the Game Plan

In the first few chapters, which you may regard as a sort of "boot camp" because you are preparing for battle, we began the journey toward achieving the health and body you have long desired. This journey will not be simple, but it will be very rewarding. Having an attractive body and tremendous energy and confidence will make people envious, wishing they had what you have, but at the same time they will be drawn to you. In addition, people in shape exude a certain healthy glow, confident energy, and a unique charisma that positively affects others around them. Suddenly, everyone wants to be just like this person in great shape. People want to look, act, and feel confident, healthy, strong, and charismatic as well. They begin asking the person in shape how he did it and if they could do it as well.

Do you understand the chain reaction? From one positive feeling to the next, everyone wants to be a part of it. Who could blame them?

Implementing the Game Plan

Prior to getting into the best shape of your life, every element must be properly placed in a specific order. I recommend organizing the meal plan and exercise regimen monthly. This way, as each month passes, goals are met. Changes will be made periodically to the diet and exercise routine in order to "shock" the body's metabolism and also to create more mental stimulation.

The first thought in your mind must be your end result—the goal you want to achieve and by when. Let us say that you want to be in the best shape by July 4th. Your motivation is that you will be attending a holiday pool party where everyone will be wearing a bathing suit. Most of your body will be exposed and you want to look good. So, your primary motivation to begin exercising and eating well is to look great that day.

But let's take it a step further. This is also your overall starting point to a healthier and better life. The party is merely what will trigger you to start exercising and eating right; short-term goals and deadlines are great motivators. The next step is the other date, namely, the date that will allow enough time for you to be in optimum shape by or before that Fourth of July pool party. Some people are content to just lose their flabby stomachs, while others just want to develop a well-defined "six-pack." This entirely depends on your goals. Using myself as an example, let's just say that on the Fourth of July I want to weigh approximately 195 pounds and have around 7 to 8 percent body fat. Currently, however, my weight is 210 pounds with 15 percent body fat. Which combination of diet and exercise will help me lose 15 pounds and lower my body fat by 7 to 8 percent? How long will it take? Given the average of losing one to two pounds and one percent of body fat per week, then an approximate amount of time needed to complete this goal would be eight weeks. We subtract two months from the Fourth of July and that equals May 4th.

Remember, however, that the more time you give yourself, the better off you will always be. The slower and more precise the meal plan and exercise regimen is, the better you will look and feel. A diet and workout regimen is something you never want to rush.

We now have the first two steps: the start and finish date. We now need to move on to step three, which is the meal plan. Choosing the proper and most effective meal plan must be carefully thought through so it matches your personal food preferences and lifestyle. It's not wise to blindly follow someone else's diet just because that particular person looks great and it worked for him. Devising your own meal plan is really what works best. Asking plenty of questions and reading many fitness magazines and articles will provide quite a bit of information for you. You could try a few different diets as a test to see which food combinations work best for you. If you hate the foods on the diet, you won't stick with it.

Trial and error may eventually work for you, but you'll waste a lot of time that way. I suggest working with a qualified personal trainer to help you get started on the right track. You still need to learn as much about nutrition as you can, because our understanding is always growing. I work hard to stay on top of current nutritional thinking. I continually update my sports nutrition knowledge because I am always looking for an edge when devising me own meal plans and the plans for my clients. I'm always learning something new that makes it easier for me to get into shape. The more I know about nutrition, the more I can maintain a good diet. Once you've educated yourself with some good nutritional knowledge, the dieting process becomes much easier. Over the years, I've experimented a lot on myself (not always successfully) to find the diet formulas that work best. I'll share them with you in this book so you can avoid some of the trial and error I went through.

For you to correctly apply step three (creating the perfect meal plan), you must first begin choosing which of the healthiest foods and the proper meal times will be most comfortable and effective for your particular taste and lifestyle. For example, if you happen to be a vegetarian, you need to make adjustments in your food choices. Another example would be your lifestyle. Is it active or sedentary? This will also affect which foods and portion sizes are best for you. What is your cultural or ethnic heritage? You want to choose foods that you like and have grown up eating. Is there a history of illness such as high cholesterol, diabetes, and/or high blood pressure in your family? Do you have these problems now? Is there a family history of cancer or any other serious illness? It's important for me to know all of this when I prepare a customized meal plan for a client. When I give nutritional advice to clients and prepare their meal plans, I take every detail into consideration: family history, fitness goals, lifestyle, and food preferences.

When all of these details are taken into account while constructing someone's diet, the success rate is much higher.

For your body to look and perform its best, eating numerous small meals is usually the most successful approach. The different meal plans I recommend in this book have worked well for me and for my clients. My primary goals in meal plans are good nutrition, simplicity, convenience, but most of all, to help you find an easier and faster way. My approach is geared toward being in shape as a long-term commitment and lifestyle.

You Are What You Eat

Preparing proper meals and knowing which foods work best for your body is an art in itself. Most people follow a diet that was either recommended for them or that they read about. Most of these diet plans claim to cause in rapid weight loss, because this is what draws everyone's attention. Most people want fast results, so they're only interested in a diet that offers just that, no matter how unhealthy the diet might be. This is a mistake. Fast-acting, short-term diets tend to fizzle out rather quickly and without achieving your desired results.

I know from many years of experience that only a carefully individualized meal plan will work for you in the long run. We need to think about what results you want to achieve. And trust me, no matter if you are overweight, normal weight, or underweight, we will devise a diet that will fit your lifestyle and help you achieve the results you desire.

I always ask my clients to get used to cooking meals at home. If you buy and cook your food yourself, then you know that every bite entering your body is carefully monitored. Prepare everything without salt—use lots of flavorful herbs and spices instead. Never fry anything. Bake, broil, steam, or lightly sauté instead.

Eating in restaurants is more of a challenge. The portions tend to be larger than is healthy. When you look at all the tempting dishes on the menu, you can easily end up skipping the best choices, such as lean meats, fish, and vegetables in favor of heavy sauces, French fries, and rich desserts. Avoid eating most prepared and fast-food meals. They're loaded with salt, added sugar, and fat.

As a general rule, I recommend following a Mediterranean style diet. A good model is the DASH diet, which is based on the Mediterranean approach of lean meats, fish, lots of fresh fruit and vegetables, and whole grains—and very little sugar. This is the proven diet doctors recommend for patients with health problems such as high blood pressure. It works even better if you don't have any chronic health problems, because this is basically a very healthy approach that will keep you feeling satisfied by your food. (To find out lots more about the DASH diet, go to the website of the National Heart, Lung, and Blood Institute, a division of the National Institutes of Health, at nhlbi.nih.gov.) Always drink plenty of plain water throughout the day. Aim for three to four quarts (8 to 12 glasses) of plain water. If you want a little variety, unsweetened iced tea or herbal tea is fine. Try to avoid sugar, including sugar from soda, fruit juice, and energy drinks. Sugar will slow down your progress by filling you with empty calories that have no nutritional value. Many fruit juices have added sugar. Stick to 100 percent natural fruit juices cut in half or even two-thirds with plain water. Artificial sweeteners are acceptable in small amounts. Bear in mind, however, that research has shown that people who drink artificially sweetened sodas gain more weight than people who drink the sugar-sweetened versions! A daily glass of red wine has numerous health benefits, but remember not to drink more than one glass. If you don't like wine, or if you need to stay away from alcohol for any reason, remember that the daily glass of wine I suggest is completely optional. If you don't want it, that's fine. I have had many clients consume red wine until intoxication, claiming they thought it would benefit them. I agree that we sometimes need to go out and have fun by having a few drinks, if that's not a problem, and eating foods that aren't part of our diets. Having some fun and a cheat meal on a weekly basis is perfectly fine and even recommended. We all need to unwind from time to time. I follow that motto!

Diets and Hormones

When people age, why do they slow down, weaken, and become frail? As we get older, the body begins to degenerate and break down. We can't stop the aging process and the body's gradual degeneration, but even as we get older we can still make the body stronger, flexible, and more toned, with less body fat. We can create our heart's desire at any age. It's all a question of how much you want it. What will be your level of dedication, drive, and commitment? It's all up to you. I have seen people in their 60s and 70s look and feel better than they ever have.

Have you ever heard people complain that their metabolisms slow down as they age? They say the have less energy, gain weight easily, don't have as much endurance as they used to. This isn't automatic. It only happens because most people live more sedate lives as they become older. Their metabolism adjusts, and as a result, slows down. This can be reversed—provided you stay active. Your body acclimates to the lifestyle you live. Because of this, it is always possible to build strength, lose body fat, and increase your energy, regardless of age. The more you commit to exercise, rest, and healthy eating, the better your body will become, because it will have more strength, endurance, and less body fat.

You are never too old and it's never too late to start changing your life for the better. People have always doubted me until seeing the results. It is all possible but you must believe in yourself. Having confidence in yourself makes achieving any dream possible. The results will not be noticed immediately, so it is very important to remain committed. Once motivated, you will begin to enjoy dieting and looking forward to achieving even a better body and health. It will seem as if you have now become addicted—in a good way—to following this new and healthy lifestyle.

When we age, our bodies experience hormonal changes that eventually lead to decreases in strength, muscle tone, and energy. Older people sleep more lightly, which also causes negative effects. Our skin loses elasticity due to decreasing levels of the body's natural production of human growth hormone (HGH). When the body's natural production of the male hormone testosterone decreases, men begin to lose physical strength, endurance, and energy. Sleeping less than seven to eight hours per night will cause the body to produce less testosterone and human growth hormone. That's because your body produces these hormones while you're sleeping. (Women also produce testosterone, just in much lower amounts.) You need to sleep seven to eight hours each night in order for the body to produce sufficient amounts of these important hormones. This is crucial, because these hormones are very important factors for anti-aging and rejuvenation.

Not sleeping enough also raises the body's level of the stress hormone cortisol. This hormone, when elevated, causes the body to consume its own muscle tissue and add to the body's fat deposit. Basically, cortisol will make you lose muscle tissue and gain body fat; if you have high cortisol levels for a long time you are more likely to develop type 2 diabetes. This is another important reason to allow the body to have adequate sleep. Cortisol is suppressed when you rest or sleep.

The proper diet is just as important as sleep for increasing the body's level of testosterone and human growth hormone. Diet and sleep improve and restore the body's natural hormone function to that of a younger person.

I stress proper nutrition for triggering the hormone response because, by having your body's endocrine (hormone) system work at its best, you are on your way to feeling and looking years younger. The key to being in fantastic shape is to follow a diet and exercise regimen that will keep your hormones working at their best possible levels.
Simply by eating properly, your facial skin will take on more of a glow and healthier look. This is part of the chain reaction that occurs once you begin following a healthier lifestyle. Once you begin following the necessary steps, your body will begin to operate like a well-oiled machine and you will feel like a new and younger person.

Chapter 6
The Diet

Phase I of my plan for rejuvenating you consisted of having the right attitude. I stressed the importance of believing in yourself and developing a winner's mentality in order to succeed. Phase II consisted of getting seven to eight hours of sleep every night to prepare yourself for maximum performance during your waking hours. Now let's move on to Phase III: your diet and moving toward eating in the healthiest possible way.

Phase III concentrates on the nutritional aspect of getting into shape. This phase will explain in detail meal options that will provide your body with the strength and energy it will need in order for you to look and feel your very best. With proper nutrition, the body will be able to reduce its body fat while adding and toning lean muscle mass.

When all three phases are in motion together, you will feel more energized and notice a substantial reduction in body fat. Please understand that the formula that I am showing you is not meant for rapid weight loss. Instead, it's designed for steady body-sculpting, meaning your body will continually transform itself into a leaner and more toned physique. This is a much more successful method than a weight-loss diet, because your body will comfortably transform without you suffering from fatigue and hunger. So-called "rapid weight-loss" programs leave you with a frail, tired, somewhat soft physique. My program will make your body firmer, toned, and stronger. Overall, you will feel much more comfortable with your new body.

Phase III

The object of phase III is to adjust your entire eating pattern. You will be eating well-balanced and well-formulated meals that will be specifically made for your particular lifestyle and taste. I don't agree with following any old diet that you've read about in a magazine, or saw on TV or the internet, or was recommended to you by someone you know. I believe your meal plan should be carefully constructed specifically for you.
Every person has an individual metabolism, personal tastes, lifestyles, and goals. Therefore, every person should have an individual meal plan as well.

Your meal plan will depend on your fitness goals and your current body type (overweight or underweight). The same principle applies to lifestyles, because some people live more active lives than others.

The foods you eat fall into three main nutritional groups: proteins, carbohydrates, and fats. Carefully combining these food groups will dictate your progress in losing fat and gaining lean muscle tissue. It is very important to understand and eventually be able to distinguish the difference and importance of each of these food groups.

<B> Protein

Protein foods contain long strings of amino acids, the building blocks of your body. Animal foods such meat, milk, cheese, eggs, and fish all contain large amounts of protein. So do some plant foods, particularly beans and nuts. Although we generally think of meat when we think of protein, it's possible to be a vegan—someone who eats no animal foods—and still get plenty of protein from your diet.

Because low-fat dairy products also contain carbohydrates in the form of lactose (the natural sugar found in milk), lean proteins are always better than dairy products when you are combining meals with other carbohydrates. Dairy products are best consumed either by themselves or combined with very small portions of either a protein or carbohydrate. Lean dairy proteins make excellent meals for weight loss if consumed by themselves.

Suggested Protein Foods

    Lean beef (eye round, London broil, other lean cuts)
    Chicken breast (skinless, boneless)
    Turkey breast (skinless, boneless)
    Lean cuts of pork
    Fish (preferably wild-caught and not farm-raised)
    Egg whites
    Protein powders (whey protein and soy protein isolate)
    Low-fat dairy products (nonfat milk, Greek yogurt, nonfat cottage cheese)

Carbohydrates

Carbohydrates are sugary or starchy foods that provide energy to the body. Your body converts carbohydrates to glucose, also known as blood sugar, which is your body's main fuel.

Carbohydrates are divided into two groups: simple and complex. Simple carbohydrates are foods that are quickly digested and absorbed into your bloodstream. Fast-acting carbs, as simple carbohydrates are also called, raise your blood sugar quickly. They're found in fruit juices, milk, and processed or refined foods such as white bread, rice, pasta, French fries, cookies, crackers, and snack foods. Simple carbohydrates work best for an energy boost without weight gain when they're consumed for breakfast and immediately after exercising.

After fasting overnight or working out, your body needs to quickly replenish its energy. Does that mean I recommend eating cookies for breakfast? No way. Instead, choose whole wheat toast, oatmeal, bran cereal with only a bit of milk, and other healthy choices that have no added sugar or fat.

Complex carbohydrates are also known as slow-burning carbs because they take longer for the body to digest and absorb. They give you a steady stream of energy instead of the quick burst from simple carbohydrates. A carbohydrate is complex when it's in its whole form and contains its natural fiber. White flour, for instance, has no fiber and so is a simple carbohydrate; whole wheat flour contains the natural bran fiber and so is a complex carbohydrate. The same is true of white rice versus brown rice. Fiber slows down the digestive process and keeps a carbohydrate food from being absorbed quickly. Fiber also helps move solid waste through the body and keeps you regular.

Suggested Carbohydrate Foods
Sweet potato, yam
Fresh fruit
Brown or wild rice
Whole-grain pasta
Whole-grain bread
Oats (not instant)
Bran
Multi-grain cereals
Whole-grain cereals
Vegetables

Simple Carbohydrates
Simple carbohydrates, also known as refined carbohydrates, enter your quickly and provide the body with instant energy. The problem with this type of carbohydrate is that it also exits the body's bloodstream quickly. That can make you feel a sudden loss of energy, as if you've run out of gas. To avoid the short-term energy burst followed by an energy crash, be sure to eat a complex carbohydrate along with a simple carb. For example, if you like to eat cereal for breakfast or a snack, be aware that milk is a simple carbohydrate. So, eat a cereal that's a complex carbohydrate, such as 100 percent bran flakes. That way you get a good mix of both quick-acting and slow-acting carbohydrates and your energy level will stay steady.

I always recommend complex carbohydrates whenever possible. Simple carbohydrates are often high in sugar and don't have much or any fiber. They're also usually highly processed, low in nutritional value, and often include added fats. There's not much good nutrition in cookies, snack foods, and French fries.

Fruits are a good source of natural carbohydrates. By fruit I mean fresh fruit with the peel (where appropriate) and no added sugar, such as is found in canned fruit and some frozen fruit. Watch out for fruit juice. It may be 100 percent natural, but juice has no fiber. That means it hits your bloodstream very quickly and can lead to a later energy crash. If you want to drink fruit juice, try cutting it with plain water, using only a few ounces of juice in a large glass. When you eat fruit, have only one piece at a time—a single banana or apple with a meal or for a snack. This keeps your blood sugar on a more even keel.

Other forms of simple carbohydrates falls under the category of refined carbohydrates, which include breads such as white bread or bagels, white rice, and potatoes, as well as any other form of highly processed foods such as pizza, donuts, cake, taco shells, most flour tortillas, sodas and fruit punches, and any other carbohydrate that is very low in fiber.

Fiber

Fiber is crucial to good health and maintaining a healthy weight. Fiber is the indigestible part of a plant food. It's mostly the cellulose that forms the cell walls of the plant—fiber is what gives a plant food its crunch. Although experts recommend getting 25 to 35 grams of fiber from your food every day, most of us get far less. Most Americans don't eat enough fruits, vegetables, and whole grains, so they don't get the fiber from these foods. To get enough fiber, you have to really apply yourself and make sure you eat enough fiber-rich foods. One good way is to trade your cookies and other snack foods for fresh fruits and vegetables; swap your sugary breakfast cereal for one with natural bran. When eating out, have a salad as an appetizer or ask for a side salad along with your main course. Trade the baked potato, pasta, fries, or rice for steamed or sautéed vegetables. Today, waiters are very used to this sort of request and will be happy to accommodate you. Whole-grain pasta, brown rice, and sweet potatoes are other good sources of fiber but usually aren't served in restaurants. If they are, take advantage of them.

One really great benefit of fiber is that it gives you that full feeling from eating, but without added calories. I've found that people who are watching their calories but not getting enough fiber tend to stagnate when it comes to weight loss. The same number of calories from foods higher in fiber gets the weight loss going again. In other words, an apple, which has about 100 calories, 4 grams of fiber, and no fat, will fill you up longer than two Oreos, which also have about 100 calories, 7 grams of fat, and no fiber. The sweet treat and crunch of the apple are much better for you in every way.

A meal with some high-fiber foods fills you up fast and keeps you feeling full longer. If you have a hamburger and fries for lunch followed by six cookies, you'll be hungry again within a couple of hours. If you have a big salad first and a piece of fruit for dessert, you probably won't be hungry again until supper time. You probably won't want that snack at 3 p.m., either. Fiber slows down the entry of glucose into your bloodstream, so you get steadier energy instead of a jolt of blood sugar followed by an energy drop and the need to eat something sugary or starchy to bring you energy level up again.

Fiber can be helpful for preventing illness. It provides a lot of bulk, so you have regular bowel movements and avoid problems such as constipation and hemorrhoids. Because fiber helps waste move through your system quickly and regularly, the walls of your intestines are in contact with waste products and any toxins for less time, which may help reduce your risk of colon cancer, which is now the number 3 cancer in the U.S.

Fiber comes in two types: soluble and insoluble. Soluble fiber absorbs water in your digestive system and expands. This makes your food move through you easily. Insoluble fiber mostly comes from pectin, the fiber found in fruits such as apples and peaches. Insoluble fiber doesn't absorb water during digestion. It provides bulk instead—think of it as broom sweeping out your intestines. It's found mostly in crunchy veggies such as celery and carrots, and in leafy green veggies such as kale, broccoli, and salad greens.

While fiber is good, too much, especially if you're not used to it, can upset your digestion and cause bloating, gas, and diarrhea. Add fiber in gradually by adding a bit more each day. If you have digestive problems, cut back a bit or stay steady until things return to normal, and then start slowly adding fiber again until you reach at least 30 grams a day.

Suggested High-Fiber Foods

Fruits
Apples
Blackberries
Blueberries
Figs
Raspberries

Vegetables
Beans
Broccoli
Cabbage
Green beans
Raspberries

Fiber Supplements
Sugar-free psyllium husk powder

Breakfast Cereals
High-fiber bran cereals
High fiber multi-grain cereals
Oat bran
Steel-cut or old-fashioned oats
Unprocessed wheat bran

When you're food shopping, look for the products that claim on the label to be high in fiber or a good source of fiber. By law, high fiber on the label means the food has 5 grams or more of fiber per serving. If the label says good source of fiber, the food has 2.5 to 5 grams of fiber per serving. Watch out for foods that say they have more or added fiber. They have at least 2.5 grams more fiber per serving than the food ordinarily has, but if it's a low-fiber or highly processed food to begin with, it's not a good choice. Watch out for foods that are high in fiber but also have added sugar—this can be a problem with many breakfast cereals. Also be careful about dried fruit. This is a good and tasty way to get fiber, but only buy products with no added sugar.

Fats

Fats make up a large part of our diet—most of us get about 35 to 40 percent of our calories from fat. Although we're told over and over by nutritionists, doctors, and everyone else that fat is bad for us, that's a very misleading message. You need fat in your diet just as much as you need vitamins. Your body uses dietary fat to make hormones (including testosterone and estrogen), to make your cell walls, to make the covering that insulates your nerves, and for energy. Your body also stores fat to cushion your organs and for energy when you've run out of blood sugar, such as when you fast overnight while you're asleep.

On the other hand, fat does have some negatives. One gram of fat has 9 calories, as opposed to calories in a gram of protein or carbohydrate, so a diet too high in fat may make you gain weight.

We need to look more closely at fat to distinguish between fats that are good for you and fats that might be harmful. Healthy fats offer tremendous benefits, such as assisting the body to maintain normal weight and maintain a healthy metabolism. They also help increase hormone levels such as testosterone and human growth hormone. Good hormone levels give you a lot of muscle-building advantages, such as helping to produce lean muscle mass, and giving you increased energy, stronger libido, and faster recovery time. A diet that contains lots of good fat also helps ward off depression.

Consuming unhealthy fats, however, causes damage to the body by increasing your bad cholesterol level. It also decreases testosterone production, which leads to decreasing muscle mass, slow metabolism, low energy levels, and possibly depression. Testosterone (and also estrogen, the female hormone) is closely related to mood. Lowered levels of these hormones can put your mind in a mentally depressed state, while higher levels can provide a happier and more positive mood. Your way of thinking has a tremendous impact on your quality of life. People who are happier also are more successful with their health and overall lifestyle.

Consuming the proper amount of healthy fats will also improve other areas of the body, such as your complexion and joint flexibility. Internally, good fats help reduce the "bad" (LDL) cholesterol and increase "good" (HDL) cholesterol. Brain function also improves, because the good fats thin the blood for better circulation. They also help improve your production of neurotransmitters, the natural chemicals your brain uses to communicate between nerves. When your brain can transport messages rapidly, your cognitive function is improved. Your memory is better and you think a bit faster. When you change your diet to improve the balance of good fats, you'll notice yourself becoming more alert, clearer thinking and faster in decision-making. A diet rich in fish, nuts, and olive oil—all good sources of healthy fats--will most definitely keep you mentally sharper, especially as you age.

Types of Fat

Good fats fall into three main categories:

Monounsaturated fat: Nuts (almonds, pistachios, cashews, peanuts, pecans, and others), avocado, olive oil, olives, canola oil, sesame seeds, peanut butter, peanut oil, grape seed oil, and flaxseed oil.

Polyunsaturated fat: Corn oil, safflower oil, soybean oil, sunflower oil, canola oil, walnuts, pumpkin seeds, sunflower seeds, walnuts and walnut oil, flaxseeds and flaxseed oil.

Omega-3 fatty acids: Walnuts and walnut oil, flaxseed and flaxseed oil, canola oil, fish oil, oily cold-water fish such as tuna, herring, mackerel, salmon, sardines. Whenever possible, choose fish and seafood that have been wild-caught, not farm-raised; these have a higher omega-3 content.

Healthy Menu with Good Fats

Breakfast	2 omega-3 eggs, using olive or canola oil spray for the pan
Snack	small handful unsalted almonds (about 10 nuts)
Lunch	1 can tuna in water, with celery and whole-grain pita bread
Snack	a few small pieces of coconut
Dinner	steamed lobster
	small sweet potato with olive oil
	vegetables with avocado

Healthy Menus with High-Quality Protein

Menu #1

Breakfast	1 cup egg whites, scrambled, using olive oil or canola spray for the pan
	1/2 cup high-fiber bran cereal with lactose-free nonfat milk
	1 banana (or fruit of your choice)
Snack	1 fruit of your choice
Lunch	4 oz. grilled chicken breast on whole-grain bread
Snack	1 small handful walnuts (about 10 nuts)
Dinner	4 oz. broiled flounder
	1 cup steamed vegetables
	sugar-free gelatin

Menu #2

Breakfast	1 scoop soy protein isolate
	1/2 cup oatmeal
	1 fruit of your choice
Lunch	1 can tuna in water
	1 cup brown rice
Dinner	broiled octopus
	1 cup whole-grain pasta with olive oil
	broiled corn on the cob
	1 cup fresh fruit cocktail

Healthy Menus with High-Quality Fat

Menu #1

Breakfast	2 omega-3 eggs, using olive oil or canola spray for the pan
	1 slice multi-grain bread with all-natural unsalted peanut butter
Snack	1 small handful walnuts (about 10 nuts)
Lunch	1 can salmon mixed with cucumbers and avocado
Dinner	6 oz. broiled eye round beef
	green salad with olive oil, balsamic vinegar, and flaxseeds
	sugar-free pudding

Menu #2

Breakfast	1 cup egg whites scrambled with organic low-fat cheese
	bran cereal with almonds
	1 fruit of your choice
Snack	1 small handful almonds (about 10 nuts)

Lunch	1 can tuna in water mixed with celery and olive oil with whole-grain pita bread
Snack	1 apple and 1 small handful walnuts (about 10 nuts)
Dinner	tofu with lemon and olive oil green salad with avocado sweet potato with olive oil 1 cup fresh fruit cocktail

Healthy Menus with High-Quality Carbohydrates

Menu #1

Breakfast	1 scoop whey protein isolate 2/3 cup old-fashioned oats mixed with blueberries
Snack	1 apple
Lunch	1 can tuna in water mixed with celery and olive oil with wild rice
Snack	1 orange
Dinner	5 oz. grilled chicken breast sweet potato steamed vegetables 1 cup sugar- and fat-free yogurt

Menu #2

Breakfast	2 whole-grain pancakes 2 soft-boiled omega-3 eggs 1 cup fresh raspberries
Snack	1 apple
Lunch	1 cup whole-grain pasta mixed with turkey breast, tomato, and cucumber with olive oil and balsamic vinegar
Snack	1 peach or fruit of your choice

Dinner   extra firm tofu mixed with brown rice vegetable soup
1 cup fresh fruit cocktail

Healthy High-Fiber Menus
Menu #1

Breakfast	2/3 cup egg whites, scrambled using olive oil or canola spray for the pan
	1 cup unprocessed wheat bran with nonfat milk
	1/2 cup fresh blueberries
Snack	1/2 cup fresh figs
Lunch	steamed shrimp with vegetables
Dinner	6 oz. London broil
	steamed cabbage
	sugar-free gelatin

Menu #2

Breakfast	1 scoop whey protein isolate
	1 cup high-fiber bran cereal with non-fat milk and figs
Lunch	extra firm tofu with broccoli
	1 high-fiber whole-grain wrap
Snack	1 cup raisins
Dinner	steamed lobster
	sautéed broccoli rabe
	1 cup fresh fruit cocktail

Meals for Overweight People
Menu #1

Breakfast	2/3 cup egg whites, scrambled using olive oil or canola spray for the pan
	1 cup oat bran with nonfat milk

Snack	1 fruit of your choice
Lunch	1 can tuna in water with lettuce, tomato, onion, and vinegar
Snack	1 small handful walnuts (about 10 nuts)
Dinner	6 oz. broiled fish
steamed carrots
sugar-free gelatin

Menu #2

Breakfast	1 scoop soy protein isolate
1 banana
Snack	1 cup nonfat Greek yogurt
Lunch	4 oz. chicken breast
cucumber and tomato salad
Snack	1 fruit of your choice
Dinner	4 oz. grilled turkey breast
steamed asparagus
1 cup fresh raspberries

Chapter 7
Different Diets for Different People

When people decide to make the choice to improve their health and body, they usually take several approaches. They read fitness books, watch health programs and videos, and ask people who are in good shape a lot of questions. Getting informed is definitely a great way to start, but you have to be willing to make modifications. The diet or fitness regimen that works well for one person may not work well for you. Everyone is different. Your personal goal might be to lose weight, or to gain weight, or to build muscle, or to be more toned, or even to prepare for a marathon. Or maybe your goal is more oriented toward your own individual health issues, such as lowering your blood pressure or your cholesterol.

Because everyone is different and has different goals, my approach to getting you into shape is very different from that of other trainers. I give you meal plans and exercise advice, but I also encourage you to experiment to find what works best for you. I place a lot of emphasis on my clients' choices and personal preferences. I spend a great deal of time listening to my clients and discussing what they want to achieve with their body and health. I need to first know what fitness goals the clients have, what types of food they like, and which workouts they enjoy. Also, I need to know about their lifestyles. In other words, I really need to develop a friendship with the client and have a lot of communication before, during, and after their fitness goals have been met.

I also think a lot about how my client can get into shape while having the most fun possible. Workouts don't have to be work. Fun is universal and everyone enjoys having a good time. Most people think of getting into shape as a painful and difficult chore. This is a big reason many either fail to improve their health or never even attempt an exercise and diet regimen. I agree that attaining a high level of fitness isn't easy. But remember my earlier discussion of quality of life? Ultimately, that's exactly what we're working to improve.

After speaking with the client, I now have an idea as to which diet and exercise routine will best fit his or her preferences and convenience. Starting with the diet, I begin constructing a meal plan that is custom-made, based on the foods the client enjoys most. Of course, the list of foods to choose from can only include healthy foods, so if your favorite food is chocolate chip cookies, you'll have to find a healthier substitute and save the cookies for a treat instead. The list of healthy foods is substantial, so you'll be able to find plenty of foods you like on it. My goal is always to make the diet as effortless as possible to maintain.

Constructing a diet that is fun to eat will increase your chances of following it. Most meal plans tend to be very bland and routine. Abiding by them becomes difficult, which causes many people to cheat on their diets, which eventually leads to the obvious, that is, not reaching the desired fitness goals. Sticking to a meal plan that you don't enjoy can be extremely difficult and ends up becoming a chore. No one wants to live that way, being obligated to eat certain foods at specific times. Constantly changing your diet is effective because it allows you to enjoy food variety, as opposed to eating the same things every day.

Check the lists below to find foods that you can incorporate into your diet. You'll see that the lists are varied and contain a lot of foods that you might not have thought of. Some of them could be considered exotic or at least a bit out of the ordinary. Keep an open mind and give the foods you've never eaten a try. I think you'll be pleasantly surprised to realize that your food doesn't ever have to be boring.

Interesting and Healthy Food Choices

Protein

Fish and seafood: lobster, squid, octopus, shrimp, clams, oysters, scallops, mussels and all others

Game meats: venison (deer), wild boar, buffalo, ostrich, emu

Carbohydrates

Fruits and vegetables: yucca, chayote, plantains, passion fruit, kiwi, Asian pear, pomegranate, persimmon

Grains: wild rice, quinoa, kasha, buckwheat noodles

Fats

Coconut and coconut oil, avocado, extra-virgin cold-pressed olive oil, nuts, olives

When people diet, they most often complain about the lack of variety with their low-calorie, healthy meals. I was one of those people. To make my meals more interesting and enjoyable, I began to research the types of foods on the menus of five-star restaurants. I wanted to increase the "fun factor" while dieting. I eat out several times a week at all sorts of different restaurants. I didn't like to order bland and boring meals such as steamed chicken and broccoli or plain grilled tuna with brown rice. These are meals that can easily be prepared at home in five minutes. I feel that by ordering dishes like that I'm wasting a night out at a beautiful restaurant. Instead, I learned how to find the healthiest and most delicious dishes on the menu. By being willing to try new dishes I get to enjoy wonderful meals made by talented chefs.

Healthy Restaurant Meals

Spanish Cuisine

Mariscada: seafood marinated in olive oil, lemon, garlic, pepper

Octopus with olive oil

Gazpacho (cold vegetable soup)

Steamed vegetables

Italian Cuisine
Shrimp cocktail
Escarole soup
Zuppa de mare (seafood stew with tomatoes)
Steamed vegetables

Greek Cuisine
Greek salad
Grilled octopus
Grilled seafood with lemon
Grilled vegetables

Chinese Cuisine
Steamed shrimp with vegetables
Stir-fried vegetables
Stir-fried tofu

Japanese Cuisine
Hibachi-grilled lobster and shrimp
Grilled *vegetables*

Steakhouse Cuisine
Garden salad (vinegar, olive oil)
Grilled mushrooms
London broil

Seafood Restaurant
Shrimp salad
Clams on the half shell
Steamed lobster
Broiled or grilled fish or shrimp
Steamed or grilled vegetables

Mexican Cuisine
Avocado salad

Chicken breast with salsa
Spicy grilled peppers

Brazilian Cuisine
Heart of palm salad
Rodizio (grilled chicken breast, lean pork and salmon)
South American Cuisine
Shrimp ceviche salad
Octopus or fish ceviche

Caribbean Cuisine
Curried chicken breast or fish
Roasted peppers and corn
Pineapple salad

Eastern European Cuisine
Beet and vegetable soup (borscht)
Cabbage salad
Boiled meat

The list of ethnic restaurants is endless, especially if you live, as I do, in a large and very diverse metropolitan region. This gives you a lot of scope for enjoying a wide range of foods while still sticking to your diet.

At any ethnic restaurant where the food might be unfamiliar, stick to these rules and you'll be sure to have an enjoyable and healthy meal:
• Always drink plenty of water. If you wish, try a mineral water from the restaurant's home country.
• Have only one glass of wine with your meal or have an after-dinner drink (if you drink before eating, you might get too relaxed and overeat or make poor food choices). Again, this is a good time to broaden your horizons by trying something different from the home country.
• Salads are found in almost every ethnic cuisine. Order a side salad

with oil and vinegar or ask for the house dressing on the side. Use it sparingly, because salad dressings tend to be high in fat and may well have added sugar.

- If you order soup, avoid anything with a creamy base. I strongly recommend ordering soup as an appetizer in an ethnic restaurants. They are always interesting and different, plus soup is a good way to cut your appetite and keep you from overeating.
- Whenever possible, order appetizers and main courses that are grilled, broiled, baked, lightly sautéed, stir-fried, or steamed. Avoid anything breaded, deep-fried, or in a heavy or creamy sauce. Look for lean cuts of beef and skinless chicken. This sounds boring, but it's not. In an Indian restaurant, for example, you can enjoy skinless tandoori chicken, which is prepared in a very hot oven with exotic spices—not something you can easily make at home.

Diets for Overweight People

Every person starts with a different body type. One person may weigh 250 pounds with 30 percent body fat, while another may weigh 200 pounds with 25 percent body fat. When it comes to improving their bodies, both people want to weigh 190 pounds and have 15 percent body fat. Both have the same goal, but because they are at different starting points, they need different diets. Another example: one person weighing 160 pounds wants to lose 5 pounds, while another person weighing 140 pounds wants to lose 10 pounds. Again, these people need to follow different programs.

On the other end of the spectrum, two people may want to gain weight, but one wants to gain more than the other. To complicate matters, some people may have only a short period of time to reach their fitness goals, while others may have more time. One person may want to look good for his wedding in four months, while another is looking further down the line and hoping to look good for a class reunion that's a year away. The point is that every person has a different goal and time frame to work within. A wise decision is to allocate more than enough time to reach your desired weight and fitness goal. Try to forget those pie-in-the-sky dreams of losing weight effortlessly and needing just a few weeks to create the body of your dreams. If you believe that's possible, you're only setting yourself up for failure.

If you're serious about achieving optimum health and a great body, you need to be in it for the long haul. You will need at a minimum several months at a comfortable pace to see positive results. Please remember that losing weight and getting into shape is like running a marathon, not a short sprint. You must choose a pace of dieting and exercising that you can comfortably maintain for months and even years.

Overweight people need to give themselves enough time to get the weight-loss and fitness process moving smoothly. Some will need more time than others, depending on their current physical condition. The process begins with understanding and accepting that the journey will be well worth it!

Often, overweight individuals have a lifestyle that revolves around food. For these people, their social lives and recreation time almost always involve some type of eating environment, such as restaurants and parties. To help you get started on the path to weight loss, change your thinking pattern of food being a big part of your entertainment. Start including other types of fun which don't include eating. Look into other activities, such as bicycle riding, playing sports, sightseeing, walking, going to movies, museums and galleries, shows—pick anything and everything you enjoy, can do alone or with others, and that doesn't include eating as the main part of the fun.

Believing in yourself will provide tremendous motivation toward taking the necessary steps to create a body you have long desired!

Diets for overweight people differ depending on such factors as the physical starting point (how overweight you are), the timeline (how much time in advance do you have to lose the weight), fitness goals (such as the desired look you want to achieve), and what types of healthy foods you most enjoy eating.

The different meals plans I list here provide a basic format for you to follow. It's important to adjust your diet as time goes on. As you lose weight and get fitter, you may need to eat more or different foods to keep your program on track. I will guide you through this process in order to make your weight-loss journey as effortless as possible.

<B>Meal Plans for Overweight People

Meals for those who are overweight should consist mostly of lean proteins and high-fiber foods, meaning lots of nonstarchy vegetables, salad, and fruit in moderation. The lean proteins should consist of egg whites, lean meats such as chicken and turkey breast, eye round beef, fish, and whey and soy protein isolates.

Never allow yourself to feel hungry—that's when people can fall of the diet and have trouble getting back on. By eating plenty of high-fiber foods, which fill you up without a lot of calories, you shouldn't be hungry. While you need to keep your protein portions measured, you can eat as many vegetables and as much salad as you want. Of course, you need to avoid vegetables in heavy cream sauces or those that breaded and deep-fried. Eat as much sautéed, grilled, or steamed zucchini as you want, but avoid fried zucchini sticks.

Food Choices for Weight Loss

Protein Choices

4 to 6 oz. chicken breast, without skin
4 to 6 oz. turkey breast
4 to 6 oz. lean beef (London broil, eye round)
4 to 6 oz. wild game such as venison
4 to 6 oz. fish (wild-caught)
1 cup egg whites
2 to 3 oz. whey protein isolate
2 to 3 oz. soy protein isolate
1 cup extra firm tofu

Fiber
all nonstarchy vegetables
salad greens
fruit, preferably higher fiber fruits such as berries, figs, apples
unprocessed wheat or oat bran

For each meal, choose one protein and one vegetable or fruit. For snacks or if you aren't feeling hungry, choose a protein portion only—a baked chicken leg, for instance. If you want a larger snack, add only salad greens or green vegetables. This is called "zeroing out," meaning that you reduce your carbohydrate intake for that meal or snack to zero by eating protein only. By consuming only protein, you make your body burn your stored fat at a faster rate.

Your body can't function properly for prolonged periods of time, however, without consuming fiber and small amounts of carbohydrates. By eliminating carbohydrate-containing high-fiber foods from one or two meals a day, you'll definitely accelerate the rate at which your body burns fat. Because your other meals throughout the day will contain fiber and some carbs, you'll burn fat in a safer way. This known as "carb rotation," meaning that you consume fiber and carbs with only some meals. To keep track, try consuming fiber-containing carbs every other meal or every third or fourth meal. Find the carb rotation pattern that leaves you feeling satisfied with your meal. This is part of fine-tuning the diet to achieve the best results and weight loss at a safe and comfortable pace.

Daily Menu Plans for Weight Loss
Menu #1
Breakfast 3/4 cup scrambled egg whites, using olive oil or canola spray for the pan
3/4 cup unprocessed wheat bran with a small amount of nonfat milk
tea or coffee

Snack	1 cup blueberries
Lunch	1 can tuna in water mixed with garden salad, olive oil and vinegar dressing
Snack	small handful walnuts (10 nuts)
Dinner	6 oz. London broil
	roasted corn on the cob
	1 cup raspberries
Snack	1 cup plain nonfat Greek yogurt

Menu #2

Breakfast	Smoothie with 2 scoops whey protein isolate blended with 1 cup blackberries, ice, and water
	tea or coffee
Snack	1 cup nonfat plain Greek yogurt
Lunch	6 oz. skinless, boneless chicken breast sautéed with 2 cups fresh or frozen vegetables, using olive oil or canola spray for the pan
Snack	1 fruit of your choice
Dinner	6 oz. grilled salmon
	garden salad with 10 almonds, olive oil, vinegar
Snack	2 hard-boiled omega-3 eggs

Daily Meatless Menu Plans for Weight Loss

Menu #1

Breakfast	1 cup nonfat plain cottage cheese
	1 banana
	tea or coffee
Snack	1/2 cup unsalted mixed nuts
Lunch	egg white omelet cooked with sliced

	tomato and spinach, using olive oil or canola spray for the pan
Snack	raw carrots and celery
Dinner	steamed lobster
	broccoli rabe steamed with garlic
	sugar-free pudding
Snack	2 hard-boiled omega-3 eggs

Menu #2

Breakfast	2 slices whole-grain toast with all-natural peanut butter
	1 scoop whey protein isolate mixed with water
	tea or coffee
Snack	1 cup canned sugar-free pineapple
Lunch	shrimp salad with lettuce, tomato, onions, olives, olive oil, vinegar
Snack	1 fruit of your choice
Dinner	sliced eye round steak grilled with onion and red pepper
	grilled corn on the cob
	sliced watermelon
Snack	2 tablespoons all-natural peanut butter

Daily Vegan Menu Plans for Weight Loss

Menu #1

Breakfast	smoothie with 2 scoops soy protein isolate blended with 1 cup blueberries, water, ice
	tea or coffee
Snack	1 fruit of your choice
Lunch	tofu salad with vegetables, olive oil, vinegar

Snack	1/2 cup unsalted mixed nuts
Dinner	tofu stir-fry with onion, pepper, garlic, broccoli
	garden salad
	sugar-free gelatin
Snack	1 fruit of your choice

Menu #2

Breakfast	8 ounces nonfat soy milk
	slice melon
	tea or coffee
Lunch	tofu steamed with broccoli rabe and served in all-natural tomato sauce
	garden salad with olives, olive oil, vinegar
	1 fruit of your choice
Dinner	1 cup wild rice mixed with 1 cup black beans
	steamed peas and Brussels sprouts
	1 cup fresh fruit cocktail
Snack	1/2 cup unsalted mixed nuts

Diets for Underweight People

People who are too thin also have concerns about their bodies. When we think about out-of-shape individuals, we usually envision people who are overweight. The reality is that there are many people who are too skinny and want to gain weight, but they don't know how to do it in healthy way. Many of the older underweight people I work with start out undernourished and very weak. Growing older is often associated with also growing weaker, because we naturally lose some muscle mass as we age. However, growing weak or even frail isn't a normal part of aging—it can and should be prevented. There's no reason for anyone to just wither away from aging alone.

Do you really want the fountain of youth? Do you really want to feel and look years younger? Because if you have the will, then I will show you the way to looking and feeling so much better! For those of you who are a little too thin and feel you could afford to add a few pounds of lean muscle, along with more strength, and better posture, then prepare yourself to follow my proven program. It begins with eating right.

One good thing about being too thin is that it lets you eat more! You actually need to consume more calories, so you never need to feel hungry. My meal plan for anyone is designed to help you avoid feeling hungry, because that makes dieting very difficult and uncomfortable. But if you're underweight, you'll really never feel hungry on my meal plan—and that will almost guarantee success.

Suggested Foods for Underweight People

Proteins
Chicken breast
Egg whites
Fish
Lean beef
Lean pork
Soy protein isolate
Turkey breast
Whey protein isolate

Carbohydrates
Brown rice
Fruit
Oats
Sweet potato
Whole-grain bread
Whole-grain pasta
Wild rice

Fats
Almonds
Avocado
Canola oil
Olive oil
Peanuts
Walnuts

Fiber
Bran
Coconut
Flaxseeds
Green vegetables
Oat bran

To effectively gain weight by adding muscle, not fat, choose one food from each food group at every meal. In combination, each food will create a balanced meal that is effective for gaining lean body mass. For example, for lunch you might have 6 ounces of broiled chicken breast (protein), along with a baked sweet potato (carbohydrate), and a large garden salad (fiber) with olive oil (fat) and vinegar dressing. That's a healthy and very satisfying meal.

Daily Menu Plans for Weight Gain
Menu #1

Breakfast	2 omega-3 eggs
	2 slices whole-grain toast with all-natural peanut butter
	1 banana
Snack	1 cup low-fat cottage cheese
Lunch	tuna in water with low-fat mayonnaise with lettuce and tomato, whole-grain pita bread
Snack	sliced cantaloupe

Dinner	6 oz. sirloin steak
	1 cup brown rice mixed with peas
	sugar-free nonfat yogurt
Snack	2 hard-boiled omega-3 eggs

Menu #2

Breakfast	scrambled egg white and low-fat cheddar cheese omelet
	sugar-free bran cereal with nonfat milk
Snack	1 fresh fruit of your choice
Lunch	tuna in water mixed with 1 cup swhole-grain pasta and olive oil
	1 fresh fruit of your choice
Snack	10 unsalted almonds
Dinner	steamed seafood combination with lemon and olive oil
	sweet potato with butter
	steamed vegetables
	fresh fruit cocktail
Snack	4 oz. grilled chicken breast

Daily Vegan Menu Plans for Weight Gain

Menu #1

Breakfast	8 ounces low-fat rice milk
	fresh fruit
Snack	1 whole-grain high-fiber wrap with all-natural peanut butter
Lunch	1 cup wild rice mixed with beans and sliced Brussels sprouts
Snack	1 fruit of your choice
Dinner	tofu stir-fried with vegetables and olive oil

	1 cup whole-grain pasta with olive oil and black pepper
	sugar-free gelatin
Snack	2 tablespoons all-natural peanut butter

Menu #2

Breakfast	smoothie with nonfat soy milk, grapes, walnuts, ice and water
Snack	1/2 cup raisins
Lunch	1 cup whole-grain pasta with all-natural tomato sauce and low-fat grated Parmesan cheese
	1 fresh fruit of your choice
Dinner	steamed tofu with onion, garlic, tomato served over wild rice
	sliced watermelon
Snack	10 almonds

Chapter 8
The Difference between Women and Men

While overall healthy eating is very important, it is even more important to know which foods work best for you. Your gender plays an important part when constructing a diet that works for you. Men and women have different metabolisms, body types, and hormones.

In general, a man's metabolism runs at a faster rate than a woman's. Men carry more muscle mass, pound for pound, compared to women; women carry more fat compared to men, even if they're not overweight. Muscle is more metabolically active than fat, so a man's metabolism will burn more calories. Man or woman, the more lean muscle mass the body carries, the more calories it will burn to maintain itself. For example, two men who both weigh 170 pounds but have different amounts of body fat will need to eat different amounts to maintain themselves. Someone with 25 percent body fat will need to eat fewer calories than someone with only 7 percent body weight. With less body fat and more lean muscle mass, the body needs more calories to nourish the extra muscle.

I often need to remind people following one of my fitness programs that they shouldn't be afraid to eat. They won't get fat as long as they eat the foods I recommend. People on diets are under the false impression that they must eat very little to improve their bodies. This isn't true at all. For the body to get into shape, you actually need to eat more food and eat more frequently—but you also have to stick to the right foods. By eating efficiently, your body's metabolism speeds up and begins to transform itself into a leaner, stronger, and better-looking physique.

Male Diet

Men should always follow a different meal plan than women. The obvious factor that men are generally larger than women and thus need more calories is only one of the reasons. A man's body almost always has more lean muscle tissue than a woman's. Lean muscle tissue requires calories in order to sustain itself, because muscle tissue consumes energy even when you're just sitting still. A muscular body will burn more calories than an overweight fat body, both during the day and even when asleep.

Hormonally, men mostly produce the male hormone testosterone, while women mostly produce the female hormone estrogen. However, men also naturally produce small amounts of estrogen, while women also naturally produce small amounts of testosterone. Testosterone helps build muscle mass, aggression, libido, and competitiveness. Because they have high levels of testosterone, men are more able to develop muscular physiques. To maintain and build their muscles, men need more food with a higher concentration of protein. Eating the proper foods will trigger an increase in a man's testosterone level, along with a decrease in estrogen. This is mostly because body fat produces estrogen in both men and women. When a man loses body fat, he produces less estrogen. This is desirable, because high estrogen levels in men can cause bloating, erectile dysfunction, and gynecomastia, which is a buildup of fatty tissue on the male breast tissue. Estrogen also causes the body to accumulate more overall body fat.

Soy foods should be eaten in moderation by both men and women, because they contain natural estrogen-like compounds that can interact with the body's estrogen receptors. In men, eating a lot of soy foods such as soy milk and tofu could increase estrogen levels and decrease testosterone levels. In women, too much soy could raise estrogen levels too high, which is a possible trigger for breast cancer and reproductive cancers. If you have ever been treated for estrogen-sensitive breast cancer or reproductive cancer, it's a good idea to eat soy only in small amounts.

Some foods can help increase a man's level of testosterone. To produce testosterone, your body needs to have a good supply of dietary fat, especially monounsaturated fats from foods such as olive oil and canola oil, polyunsaturated fats from nuts, fish oil, and flaxseed oil, and saturated fats from red meat, eggs, and dairy products. By making sure to eat enough dietary fat, you will naturally raise your body's testosterone production. Dietary fats are also helpful for reducing inflammation. Among other things, reducing inflammation reduces aches and pains, increases blood flow, and improves cognitive function. The fats and sugar in most processed and fried foods actually cause inflammation and make your blood thicker, which impairs good blood flow to the body and brain.

Female Hormones
A woman's body and internal hormonal structure is quite different than a man's. There is usually a higher body fat content in a woman's body, because the extra body fat is needed in order for their effective internal hormonal function. Among the major differences between the male and female body is the woman's naturally higher level of the female hormone estrogen. Women do also have very low levels of the male hormone testosterone, just as men have very low levels of estrogen. As women age and pass through menopause, they slowly and naturally stop producing much estrogen. This is a normal process that has some impact on your ability to build muscle. To help counter some of the normal side effects of estrogen loss, such as thinning hair, vaginal dryness, and bone loss, women can consider adding foods that are high in phytoestrogens (natural chemicals that weakly imitate estrogen) to their diet. Good choices are a soy foods such as soy protein isolate, soy milk, and tofu. However, women who have had breast or reproductive cancer or who are at risk for these cancers should not add large amounts of soy foods to the diet. Small amounts no more than a few times a week are generally safe for most women.

Females must consume a slightly different diet than males. Their diet needs to contain lower amounts of protein, simply because of their lower amount of lean muscle mass. Aside from a lower amount of protein, they also require fewer overall calories. A woman's metabolism is slightly slower because of her naturally lower amount of lean body muscle mass. The more muscle tissue the body has, then the more calories will be needed to maintain it.

Foods that Increase Testosterone

For the body and brain to perform at their best, add these anti-inflammatory and testosterone-increasing foods to your daily diet:

    Lean red meat
    Monounsaturated fats from nuts, olive oil, and canola oil
    Saturated fats in small amounts from red meat, eggs, and dairy products

Foods that Are Anti-Inflammatory

    Polyunsaturated fats from fish, fish oil, flaxseeds, flaxseed oil, and nuts
    Vegetables, especially dark green leafy vegetables
    Red wine in moderation
    Monounsaturated fats from peanuts, peanut oil, almonds, olives, olive oil, and canola oil

Daily Meal Plans for Men

Menu #1

Breakfast	2 omega-3 eggs
	8 to 10 unsalted almonds
	1 fresh fruit of your choice
Snack	1 tablespoon all-natural peanut butter
Lunch	1 can salmon with garden salad
Snack	1 fresh fruit of your choice
Dinner	6 oz. London broil
	vegetables with olive oil
	sugar-free gelatin with walnuts

Snack	1 fruit of your choice

Menu #2

Breakfast	1 scoop whey protein isolate shake blended with 8 almonds
	1/2 cup oats blended with ice, water, fruit
Snack	1/2 cup raisins
Lunch	steamed shrimp with mixed vegetables, nuts
	1 fruit of your choice
Snack	1 high-fiber English muffin with all-natural peanut butter
Dinner	grilled lobster, shrimp, onion and garlic
	garden salad with nuts, olive oil, olives and vinegar
	fresh fruit cocktail with cashews
Snack	10 almonds

Daily Meal Plans for Male Weight Loss

Menu #1

Breakfast	1 cup egg whites, scrambled
	1 cup sliced kiwi or fresh fruit of your choice
Snack	1 cup nonfat plain Greek yogurt
Lunch	6 oz. grilled turkey breast with tomato, lettuce, onion, vinegar, olive oil
Snack	sliced carrots and celery with nonfat mayonnaise
Dinner	6 oz. grilled eye round beef sautéed with vegetables
	grilled corn on the cob
	sliced coconut

Snack	1/2 cup raisins

Menu #2 (meatless)

Breakfast	2 omega-3 eggs, hard-boiled
	1 cup low-fat plain cottage cheese
Snack	1/2 cup raisins
Lunch	sautéed octopus with olive oil and onion
	steamed vegetables
Snack	1 scoop whey protein isolate blended in water
Dinner	6 oz. broiled fish with lemon
	avocado and onion salad
	1 cup red grapes or fresh fruit of your choice

Menu #3 (vegan)

Breakfast	smoothie made with 12 oz. nonfat rice milk blended with 1 banana, water, ice
Snack	1 apple or fruit of your choice
Lunch	12 oz. nonfat rice milk
	garden salad with walnuts and olive oil
Snack	1 scoop nonfat hemp protein mixed with water
Dinner	sautéed tofu with peas, broccoli, red pepper, olive oil, onion
	sliced watermelon and kiwi
Snack	1/2 cup raisins

Hormone-Boosting Meals for Underweight Males

Menu #1

Breakfast	2 omega-3 eggs scrambled with low-fat cheese

	2 oatmeal pancakes (made with honey, oats, low-fat milk)
Snack	1 cup sliced pineapple or fresh fruit of your choice
Lunch	cheeseburger made with 6 oz. lean ground beef, low-fat cheese, mustard, sliced tomato, onion, on a whole-grain bun
Snack	1 pickle
Dinner	roasted lean pork loin cooked with sweet potato, red pepper, onion, garlic, black pepper, lemon
	low-fat sugar-free ice cream
Snack	2 hard-boiled omega-3 eggs

Menu #2

Breakfast	protein shake made with 8 walnuts, 1/2 cup oatmeal, 1 scoop whey protein isolate, 1 banana, water, ice
Snack	1 cup low-fat plain Greek yogurt
Lunch	2 low-fat turkey hotdogs on whole-grain buns, low sodium sauerkraut, chili beans
Dinner	6 oz. sautéed turkey breast with broccoli rabe, garlic, and olive oil
	1 cup whole-grain pasta
Snack	1/2 cup raisins

Menu #3 (meatless)

Breakfast	egg white omelet with spinach, low-fat cheese
	1 cup oatmeal with blueberries

Snack	1/2 cup unsalted nuts
Lunch	tuna in water mixed with 1 cup brown rice and peas
	1 banana or fruit of your choice
Snack	1 cup low-fat pineapple cottage cheese
Dinner	BBQ salmon with lemon, black pepper
	BBQ roasted sweet potato
	BBQ roasted corn on the cob
	sugar-free chocolate pudding
Snack	2 hard-boiled omega-3 eggs

Menu #4 (meatless)

Breakfast	1 cup low-fat blueberry Greek yogurt
	2 omega-3 hard-boiled eggs
	1 high-fiber English muffin with 1 tablespoon all-natural peanut butter
Snack	1 fruit of your choice
Lunch	6 oz. grilled served in a high-fiber whole-grain wrap with sliced tomato, onion, vinegar, lemon
Dinner	steamed lobster with lemon
	1 cup whole-grain pasta with olive oil, black pepper, garlic
	baked vegetables with low-fat grated cheese

Menu #5 (vegan)

Breakfast	smoothie made with 1 cup nonfat rice milk, sliced banana, 2 tablespoons all-natural peanut butter, 1/2 cup oats, water, ice
Snack	1 high-fiber English muffin with 2 tablespoons almond butter

Lunch	1 cup wild rice mixed with 1 cup navy beans and onion
	sliced melon
Snack	1 cup red grapes or fruit of your choice
Dinner	tofu baked with tomato, onion, sweet potato, black pepper
	sugar-free gelatin
Snack	1 cup nonfat rice milk

Menu #6 (vegan)

Breakfast	2 slices whole-grain wheat bread with 2 tablespoons all-natural peanut butter, 2 teaspoons preserves
Snack	1 fruit of your choice
Lunch	green salad with lettuce, tomato, almonds, walnuts, tofu, cucumber, onion, olive oil, vinegar
Dinner	vegetable paella (wild rice cooked with tomato, garlic, string beans, peas, black beans, red pepper)
	sautéed string beans (olive oil, pepper)
	fresh fruit cocktail
Snack	1/2 cup raisins

Chapter 9
Feeling the Difference

Maximizing your body's hormones will quickly make you feel different—in a good way! Eating hormone-enhancing meals will immediately and effectively make positive changes in your body. Your higher hormone levels will give the body more physical energy and drive. Mentally, you'll begin to feel more focused, up-beat, and determined. Everything about you will change for the better.

In my opinion, nutritionists and trainers don't place enough importance on maximizing the body's natural hormone production. For example, when an athlete begins to decline in his performance, it's quickly blamed on being too old or "washed up." It's more likely that the athlete isn't training or dieting as efficiently and as intensely as he did when he was younger. So why isn't he training or dieting as intensely now? Most likely, it's because he has lost the drive and the motivation he had earlier. Why was this lost? His level of testosterone has decreased, leading to decreased energy, aggression, motivation, competitiveness, and drive. Testosterone decreases naturally beginning in your 30s, when the "old" or "washed-up" factor begins to occur. You begin losing that zest for life, that fire and will to win. However, this process either doesn't have to occur or it can be drastically slowed down by simply adjusting your body's sleep pattern, diet, and workout regimen.

Start by sleeping eight hours a night. When you sleep, your body does its natural repairs and releases growth hormone, which in turn helps increase your production of testosterone.

Proper training also improves the body's hormone production. When you follow a pattern of resistance training and rest time, your body triggers itself to produce more testosterone. Good nutrition is another factor, because the amount of good fats you eat can have a drastic effect on increasing your natural hormone levels.

Combining All Three

Now let's combine the first three of the four phases of getting into shape. The first phase was psychology, meaning that first you must prepare your mind to make beneficial life changes. The second phase includes sleep. For your body to effectively lose body fat, gain lean muscle mass, and be fully energized you must have adequate sleep each night, usually seven to eight hours. The third phase is dedicated to nutrition, meaning selecting foods that will bring your body to the next level in fitness and health. Phases one, two and three work together, because once your mind is prepared and focused, you can then make the changes that let you be sure to get enough sleep each night and stick to your meal plan.

Food for Females

When I work with a woman to design a meal plan, I have to take different factors into consideration than when I design a plan for a man. These factors include the woman's fitness goals and timeline, her current body weight, her age, and her food preferences. We need to consider if she prefers a specific dietary approach, such as veganism (no animal foods) or just has some particular foods she can't eat due to food allergies or dislikes. We also look at her lifestyle to see how physically active she is, what her social life is like, what she enjoys doing, and so on. If she is approaching or is past menopause, we may look into ways to add natural estrogen to her diet, as long as that's safe for her (no history of breast or reproductive cancer).

Once we've considered all the factors, I then customize a specific meal plan that will work most effectively. My main priority when working with clients is for them to achieve results. This is why I customize their diets; it will increase their chances of success.

Hormone-Boosting Diet for Women

Menu #1

Breakfast	1 omega-3 egg
	1/2 cup oatmeal with flaxseeds
Snack	1 cup blueberry nonfat Greek yogurt
Lunch	tuna in water with low-fat mayonnaise and celery
	12 oz. nonfat soy milk
Snack	1 fruit of your choice
Dinner	5 oz. grilled fish
	1 cup whole-grain pasta with olive oil, nonfat cheese
	garden salad with tofu, olives, olive oil, vinegar
Snack	1 hard-boiled omega-3 egg

Menu #2

Breakfast	scrambled egg whites
	bran cereal with nonfat soy milk
	1 banana or fruit of your choice
Snack	½ cup walnuts and almonds
Lunch	5 oz. grilled chicken breast on whole-grain rye bread
	1 cup brown rice
	12 oz. nonfat soy milk
Dinner	sautéed tofu with mixed green vegetables, olive oil
	1 sweet potato with olive oil
	garden salad with flaxseeds, olive oil, vinegar

sugar-free gelatin
Snack   1/2 cup raisins

Weight-Loss Diet for Women

Menu #1

Breakfast	high-fiber sugar-free bran cereal with nonfat soy milk and fresh blueberries
Snack	zero-calorie iced tea
Lunch	4 oz. cooked turkey breast with vegetables in a high-fiber, low-carb whole-grain wrap
Snack	1 peach or fruit of your choice
Dinner	baked tofu with tomatoes and onion
	steamed kale and garlic
	sliced fresh strawberries
Snack	10 almonds

Menu #2

Breakfast	1/2 cup egg white omelet
	1 cup fresh watermelon or fruit of your choice
Snack	raw vegetables with nonfat dip
Lunch	4 oz. lean hamburger on whole-grain bun
	garden salad with flaxseed oil, vinegar
	1 cup sliced pineapple or fruit of your choice
Snack	10 almonds
Dinner	5 oz. BBQ fish
	tofu salad (greens, tofu, olives, tomato, onion, canola oil, vinegar)
	1 kiwi fruit or fruit of your choice
Snack	1/2 cup raisins

Menu #3 (meatless)

Breakfast	1/2 cup oatmeal mixed with 1 scoop of soy protein isolate
Snack	zero-calorie iced tea or other flavored beverage
Lunch	1 can octopus garden salad, olive oil, vinegar
Snack	1 pear or fruit of your choice
Dinner	boiled seafood combination (lobster, shrimp, scallops) broccoli fresh fruit cocktail with sugar-free whipped cream
Snack	12 oz. nonfat soy milk

Menu #4 (meatless)

Breakfast	2 omega-3 scrambled eggs 1 banana or fruit of your choice
Snack	10 almonds
Lunch	tuna in water with steamed vegetables, low-fat mayonnaise in a whole-grain wrap
Dinner	BBQ fish BBQ red peppers sugar-free nonfat soy pudding
Snack	1/2 cup raisins

Menu #5 (vegan)

Breakfast	1/2 cup oat bran mixed with 1 scoop soy protein isolate and blueberries
Snack	1 soy protein bar
Lunch	12 oz. nonfat soy milk 1 apple or fruit of your choice

Snack	10 almonds
Dinner	tofu simmered in tomato sauce and broccoli
	lentil soup
	sugar-free gelatin
Snack	1/2 cup raisins

Menu #6 (vegan)

Breakfast	smoothie made with 1 scoop soy protein isolate, banana, walnuts, water, ice
Snack	sliced cantaloupe or fruit of your choice
Lunch	wild rice mixed with beans and peas
	raw vegetables nonfat vegetable dip
Snack	10 almonds
Dinner	baked beans mixed with vegetables and tofu
	steamed cabbage with spicy mustard
	fresh strawberries with sugar-free whipped soy cream
Snack	1/2 cup raisins

Weight-Gain Diet for Women

Menu #1

Breakfast	2 omega-3 scrambled eggs with low-fat cheese
	2 high-fiber waffles with sugar-free syrup
	12 oz. nonfat soy milk
Snack	1 soy protein bar
Lunch	6 oz. lean beef burger with low-fat cheese, tomato, pickle on whole-grain bun

Snack	1 kiwi fruit or fruit of your choice
Dinner	BBQ chicken breast with lemon
	sweet potato with low-fat cheddar cheese
	Greek salad
	low-fat sugar-free ice cream with walnuts
Snack	10 almonds

Menu #2

Breakfast	egg white, spinach, and low-fat cheese omelet
	1 cup soy nuts cereal with nonfat soy milk
	1 banana or fruit of your choice
Snack	1/2 cup unsalted mixed nuts
Lunch	5 oz. grilled turkey breast with olive oil
	1 cup wild rice mixed with 1 cup corn kernels
Dinner	6 oz. London broil
	grilled peppers
	1 cup whole-grain pasta with olive oil
	1 cup red grapes or fruit of your choice
Snack	1/2 cup raisins

Menu #3 (meatless)

Breakfast	egg white omelet with tomato and low-fat cheese
	1 high-fiber English muffin with all-natural peanut butter and all-natural fruit preserves
Snack	12 oz. nonfat soy milk
Lunch	1 can salmon mixed with 1 cup whole-

	grain pasta, 1 cup corn kernels, olive oil, black pepper
Snack	1 soy protein bar
Dinner	6 oz. baked fish with tomato, onion, sweet potato
	garden salad with tofu and flaxseed oil
	1/2 cup soy nuts
	1 cup raspberries
Snack	1/2 cup raisins

Menu #4 (meatless)

Breakfast	2 soft-boiled omega-3 eggs
	2 high-fiber pancakes
	12 oz. nonfat soy milk
Snack	1 orange or fruit of your choice
Lunch	Chinese-style steamed shrimp with vegetables
	1 cup wild rice
	12 oz. nonfat soy milk
Snack	10 almonds
Dinner	broiled lobster
	octopus salad
	baked sweet potato
	sautéed broccoli rabe
	sugar-free soy pudding
Snack	1/2 cup raisins

Menu #5 (vegan)

Breakfast	smoothie made 12 oz. nonfat soy milk, 10 almonds, 1 banana, 1/2 cup oats, ice
Snack	1 sugar-free frozen fruit pop
Lunch	lentil soup

	1 cup brown rice mixed with 1/2 cup kidney beans, sliced carrots, cauliflower
Snack	12 oz. nonfat soy milk
Dinner	tofu stir-fried with garlic, lemon, spinach, olive oil, flaxseeds, tomato, broccoli
	baked sweet potato
	sliced cantaloupe or fruit of your choice
Snack	1/2 cup raisins

Menu #6 (vegan)

Breakfast	whole-grain bagel with all-natural peanut butter
	1 cup blueberries mixed with 10 unsalted cashew nuts
	12 oz. nonfat soy milk
Snack	1 soy protein bar
Lunch	shake with 1 scoop soy protein isolate, 1 tablespoon all-natural peanut butter, 1 banana, 1/2 cup oats, water, ice
Snack	10 almonds
Dinner	tofu with 1 cup whole-grain pasta, olive oil, flaxseeds, black pepper
	sautéed green beans with olive oil, peppers, onion
	1 cup red grapes or fruit of your choice
Snack	1/2 cup raisins

Chapter 10
Meal Frequency and Portions

Eating well-balanced meals is an absolute necessary step for the body to achieve its maximum results. Consuming healthy meals will help your body make substantial positive changes. You will immediately feel more energized and have a feeling of lightness, as though you had already lost a few pounds of unwanted body fat. Your skin will also have a healthier glow and a more youthful and fresher look. Internally, you body will begin to cleanse itself of impurities and toxins.

Eating a healthier diet is only the first part of two-part process. The second part is meal frequency. Knowing exactly when to eat is just as important as knowing what to eat. Your body can digest only a moderate amount of food at any given time of the day. On average, your food can be most efficiently digested if you eat approximately every two to four hours. Have you ever noticed that newborn babies need to eat every two to four hours as well? This is because their digestive system works effectively, enabling the body to receive a constant flow of nutrients. Unfortunately, most people tend to eat full meals two or three times per day. Because you get hungry between meals, you end up eating larger portions at meals, both because you're hungrier and because you know it will be several hours before your next meal. Your body adjusts to the typical meal schedule by slowing down to conserve energy and make it last until the next meal. Your body goes into efficiency mode and burns fewer calories overall throughout the day, making it more difficult for you to lose body fat. In efficiency mode, the body will tend to store as much fat as possible as a way to have an energy reserve. When your body isn't receiving food frequently enough, your metabolism slows so you consume fewer overall calories. The calories you don't burn get stored as energy, otherwise known as body fat.

When and What To Eat?

For your body to function most efficiently, it is best to consume smaller portions of food more frequently throughout the day. On average, each meal should contain approximately 30 to 35 grams of protein, 35 to 40 grams of complex carbohydrates, and 5 to 10 grams of healthy monounsaturated and polyunsaturated fats. Saturated fats should be kept to at a minimum and trans fats (also called partially hydrogenated vegetable oil) should be avoided completely.

The size of the meal portions will vary from person to person, and also for each person as time goes on. For example, those who want to lose weight need a diet with a lower carbohydrate and higher protein content. Those who are looking to gain lean body mass need to consume more fats and complex carbohydrates. Another factor that needs to be taken into consideration is the individual's lifestyle, meaning his or her activity level throughout the day. Between their jobs and favorite activities, some people live very active lives, while others are more sedentary. These factors come in to play when constructing a particular diet for a specific individual.

I recommend a meal frequency that gets away from one or two big meals a day. Instead, I suggest consuming moderate amounts of food at regular intervals throughout the day. I also suggest adjusting your meal times to work with your personal appetite schedule. Some people are hungrier at certain times of the day and feel less hungry at others. You might not usually feel very hungry when you wake up, but someone else might always wake up feeling ravenous. This is perfectly normal.

During those times of the day when you feel hungriest, I suggest eating more frequently. Your portion size will stay the same. You'll be eating more often, but not more. If you feel very hungry between noon and 4 p.m., for instance, then eat a small meal every 90 minutes or two hours. This will effectively satisfy your body's need for more food and keep you from overeating later on. If, on the other hand, you're not usually very hungry during those hours, you can reduce your meal frequency to every three or four hours.

Meal Timing

The main objective of having well-timed, frequent meals is for your body to receive a steady stream of nutrients continually throughout the day. The food you eat at a meal will fuel your body for a few hours. If too long a time passes between meals, your body's metabolism will begin to slow down to conserve energy. When this occurs, instead of burning extra calories, your body stores them as fat. This keeps you from building muscles and may even cause you to lose muscle if you go for too long between meals. I see this with clients who are used to eating lightly during the day, sometimes even skipping lunch, and eating a large evening meal. Until we adjust their meal frequency to give them a steady intake of fuel throughout the day, they have trouble losing weight or building muscles. When my clients begin to eat frequently, usually every two to four hours, they begin to see results.

You'll know when it's time to eat because you'll begin to feel hungry and notice that your stomach is rumbling. Your body is signaling for more food. It's important to respond to the signal quickly. If you ignore your hunger signal, I can almost guarantee that you'll overeat at your next meal. If you listen to your body, you'll never get so hungry that you overeat. You'll be able to stick to smaller portions and you'll be less inclined to cheat on your diet. Your body and health will see the best results simply by eating smaller but well-balanced meals four to six times per day.

If you want to eat six meals a day, you might start with breakfast at 6 a.m., have a mid-morning snack at 9 a.m., lunch at noon, a mid-afternoon snack at 3 p.m., dinner at 6 p.m., and a late-night snack at 9 p.m. For five meals a day, start with breakfast at 7 a.m., and have snacks and meals every three hours after that, but skip the late-night snack. For only four meals a day, eat breakfast at 7 a.m., lunch at 1 p.m., a snack at 4 p.m., and dinner at 7 p.m. Skip the late-night snack.

Proper Portions

Consuming the right meal portions is extremely important. Most people are under the impression that as long as they eat healthy food, they will remain healthy and never be overweight. This is not true at all. Healthy foods are necessary, but that doesn't mean you can eat them in unlimited amounts. Consuming the proper quantity of food during each meal is what will really make the difference in your physique. Portion control is how you lose unwanted body fat and gain lean muscle tissue.

Consuming too much food at one time will lead to unwanted weight gain, even if the meal is healthy, such as chicken breast and baked sweet potato. One moderate portion of chicken and one medium sweet potato is fine; anything more than that, however, will keep you from attaining your goal.

We often eat until we feel full. This is definitely the wrong approach. Your stomach is similar to a balloon, because it stretches or shrinks according to the quantity of food you put into it. When you continually eat until you feel full, the stomach stretches to accommodate the extra food. After time and time again of eating until you are beyond satisfied, your stomach becomes almost permanently stretched out and enlarged. Once it is enlarged, you will need to eat larger food portions, not to give yourself enough fuel but just to not feel hungry. By consuming more food at each meal, you eventually gain weight, even when you eat foods that are low in calories and are healthy choices. Too much of a good thing can be bad.

You need to think carefully about your portions and take in the right serving size at each meal. Simply by eating the proper amount for each meal, you will quickly notice a difference. After a meal, you'll feel energized, instead of sluggish from overeating. The human body can only digest a certain amount of food at one time and anything more will eventually convert to body fat. Each individual varies, but on average the body can digest up to 25 to 35 grams of protein, up to 45 grams of carbohydrates, and 10 grams of fat from a meal. Depending on your weight, age, and activity level, these amounts can vary somewhat. During certain times of the day, your body may need more or less food from meal. For breakfast and after working out, for example, you will need to eat a larger meal. Later in the evening, you will probably need a smaller meal or snack.

Meal Portion Size

When people eat, they only rarely consider the meal's portions and the amount of protein, carbohydrates, and fat it contains. We can measure the amount of the food to determine its nutritional contents in two different ways: by weight or by quantity. To measure weight, you need to use a simple, inexpensive food scale. To measure quantity, you can use standard measuring cups and spoons.

As the weight and quantity of a food increases, so does the nutritional content. What is the proper weight and quantity of food that will equal the amount of protein, fat, and carbohydrates that your body needs for your current fitness goals? As each ounce of food increases, so do the amount of nutrients. For example, if you want to prepare a meal that has 35 grams of protein, you need to know that an ounce of meat of any sort has about 7 grams of protein. So, divide 35 by 7 and you get 5. That means 5 ounces of chicken breast, fish, or beef will have about 35 grams of protein. Use your food scale to weigh out the right amount.

If you wanted to eat 40 grams of carbohydrates for breakfast, you need to know that an ounce of a food such as oatmeal has about 4 grams of carbohydrates. So, if you wanted to eat 40 grams of carbohydrates, you would need eat about 10 ounces of oatmeal. You can use a measuring cup to measure out about two-thirds of a cup, or you can use your food scale to weigh out 10 ounces.

If you want to eat 7 grams of fat—from olive oil, for instance—measure out 1 tablespoon. After a while, you'll be able to eyeball the right amounts and won't need to measure or weigh so often. It's still important to keep an eye on your portions so you don't end up eating more than you realize. When you eat a packaged or prepared food, be sure to check the food facts label to make see what the portion size is. You might be tempted to eat the entire package or container, but that might well give you two or even more portions for that food.

You may be surprised by what a difference eating measured portions will make. Just a couple of extra ounces in a portion can make or break the look of your entire physique.

Adjusting Portion Sizes

Depending on your fitness goals, your portion sizes and ratios will vary. If you want to lose weight, you'll need to decrease your carbohydrate portions. If you want to gain weight, you'll need to increase the fat and carbohydrate content in each meal you consume. Check the chart below to see how to adjust your portions of protein, fat, and carbohydrates to achieve your goal.

Portion Adjustments

To lose body fat and weight, each meal should contain:

Protein	35-40 grams
Carbohydrates	30-35 grams, primarily from vegetables and fruit
Fat	up to 10 grams

To gain weight and lean muscle tissue, each meal should contain:

Protein	30-35 grams
Carbohydrates	45-55 grams, primarily from vegetables and fruit
Fat	5-10 grams

Chapter 11
Carbohydrates and Fast Weight Loss

The dieting method known as "carbohydrate depletion" or "carbohydrate alternation" can be an effective way to lose weight quickly. This works by alternating the amount of carbohydrates you eat. For the first three days of the week, you eat very few carbohydrates. For the next three days, you eat more carbs. The final day of the week is your "cheat" day, meaning that you can eat whatever food you want in whatever portions you want on that day—and only that day.

The purpose of carb depletion is to help you lose body fat at a faster rate. While you follow this program, your body will rid itself of excess water during the low-carb days. During the carb-loading days, your muscles will retain water and expand. This tightens the skin in order to accommodate the now larger muscle. Your body gets a tighter and leaner look.

The typical carb depletion cycle usually last several weeks. It's simplest to begin the weekly cycle on a Monday and complete it with your cheat day on a Sunday. On Monday, Tuesday, and Wednesday, your carb depletion days, you may feel somewhat tired and hungry. On Thursday, Friday, and Saturday, your carb loading days, you will probably feel energized; your muscles will feel more full and tight.

Carbohydrate rotation works because after dieting for a while, your body begins to lower its metabolism in response to your lower calorie intake. When this occurs, the rate at which your body consumes its own fat begins to slow down. Your body hits the wall, meaning it reaches a weight-loss plateau. You no longer notice any more improvement and body fat loss. Alternating your carbohydrate intake prevethis from occurring.

While you are on the carb rotation diet, be sure to eat every 3 to 4 hours. You may have coffee and tea; use artificial sweetener. If you wish, you may have one glass of red or white wine with dinner. Drink plenty of water throughout the day: three to four quarts a day.

Cheat Days

On your Sunday (or whatever day you choose) cheat day, you may eat any food you desire, even pizza, French fries, pancakes, butter, fried chicken, cake, and ice cream. On a cheat day, you not only eat any food you want in whatever quantities you want, you eat them whenever you want. The purpose of having a cheat day is to physically shock your system by feeding your body high-calorie, high-carb foods. You also give yourself a mental break by allowing yourself to eat the foods you've been craving all week. By allowing a day off from your diet, you will have a much easier time maintaining your diet and will be more successful in achieving your fitness goals.

What to Drink

Be sure to drink plenty of plain water throughout the day. I recommend three to four quarts (8 to 12 glasses) daily. You can also drink unsweetened iced tea or herbal tea or 100 percent fruit juice thinned with plain water. Avoid beverages with added sugar, such as soda, energy drinks, and fruit juice. Keep artificially sweetened drinks to a minimum. Coffee and tea are fine, but avoid adding milk or sugar to them. If you wish, one glass of red or white wine with dinner is acceptable. Wine is optional, however, and you should feel free to skip it if you prefer or if you are concerned about the effects of alcohol on you.

Carbohydrate Rotation Menus

Lower carbohydrate days: Monday, Tuesday, Wednesday
Higher carbohydrate days: Thursday, Friday, Saturday
Cheat day: Sunday

Monday, Tuesday, Wednesday nutrient goals
Protein
35 grams per meal
Carbohydrates
minimal amounts from nonstarchy vegetables and some
 fruit only
Fat
up to 10 grams per meal

Monday menu
Breakfast
1 cup egg whites scrambled with 1 omega-3 egg,
 1 fresh fruit of your choice
Snack
1 cup plain, nonfat Greek yogurt
Lunch
5 oz. skinless chicken breast with lettuce, tomato, onion,
 pepper, carrots, olive oil, vinegar
Snack
chopped raw vegetables (celery, carrots)
Dinner
6 oz. lean beef
garden salad
steamed cabbage

Tuesday menu
Breakfast
1 1/2 scoops of whey or soy protein isolate blended with 1
 fresh fruit, water, ice
Snack
1 cucumber or pickle
Lunch
5 oz. grilled turkey breast

red cabbage and beet salad
Snack
1 fresh fruit of your choice
Dinner
6 oz. steamed chicken breast with Asian vegetables

Wednesday menu
Breakfast
1 cup egg whites scrambled with 1 whole omega-3 egg
Snack
1 fresh fruit of your choice
Lunch
1 can tuna in water mixed with lettuce, onion, olives, olive oil, vinegar
Snack
1 fresh fruit of your choice
Dinner
BBQ 6 oz. lean steak
BBQ peppers and corn on the cob

Thursday, Friday, Saturday nutrient goals
Protein
30 grams
Carbohydrates
30-40 grams
Fat
up to 5 grams

Thursday menu
Breakfast
3/4 cup egg whites, scrambled
1 cup sugar-free bran cereal with nonfat milk
Snack
1 low-fat granola bar

Lunch
lean burger on a whole-grain bun
12 oz. nonfat milk
Dinner
6 oz. lean pork
1 cup whole-grain pasta with nonfat cheese
steamed broccoli

Friday menu
Breakfast
1 scoop whey or soy protein isolate with water
1 cup oatmeal
1 banana
Snack
1 low-fat protein bar
Lunch
chicken breast sandwich on rye bread
1 cup wild rice with chopped broccoli
Snack
1 fresh fruit of your choice
Dinner
5 oz. BBQ fish
baked sweet potato
garden salad, olive oil, vinegar

Saturday menu
Breakfast
1 cup egg whites, scrambled
2 high-fiber pancakes
Snack
1 fresh fruit of your choice
Lunch
5 oz. grilled salmon

steamed vegetables
brown rice
Snack
1 low-fat protein bar
Dinner
sautéed turkey breast with garlic
Greek salad
whole grain pasta with olive oil and red pepper

Meatless Carbohydrate Rotation Menus

Monday menu

Breakfast	1 scoop whey or soy protein isolate blended with 8 almonds, water, ice
Snack	1 fresh fruit of your choice
Lunch	1 can tuna in water with sliced celery, carrots, onion, vinegar
Snack	1/2 cup unsalted nuts or 1 fresh fruit of your choice
Dinner	6 oz. broiled salmon with lemon and capers
	lentil and vegetable soup
	Greek salad

Tuesday menu

Breakfast	egg white and vegetable omelet
	1 fresh fruit of your choice
Snack	1 low-fat, low-carb protein bar
Lunch	steamed shrimp with mixed vegetables
Snack	melon slices
Dinner	steamed lobster with lemon
	corn on the cob

Wednesday menu

Breakfast	1 cup plain Greek nonfat yogurt
	fresh blueberries
Snack	sliced pickles
Lunch	canned octopus
	garden salad
Snack	watermelon slices
Dinner	1/2 dozen clams on the half shell
	6 oz. baked fish
	tomato, onion, and olive salad

Thursday menu

Breakfast	sugar-free high-fiber bran cereal with nonfat milk
	1 scoop whey (men) or soy (women) protein isolate mixed with water
Snack	1 hard-boiled egg with whole-grain toast
Lunch	Chinese-style steamed shrimp and vegetables
	brown rice
Snack	1 kiwi fruit
Dinner	6 oz. baked scrod with tomato
	sweet potato

Friday menu

Breakfast	2 hard-boiled omega-3 eggs
	1 high-fiber English muffin
Snack	1 pear
Lunch	sautéed shrimp with red pepper, olive oil
	1 cup wild rice
Snack	12 oz. low-fat milk (men) or soy milk (women)

Dinner	broiled clams and scallops with olive oil and lemon
	1 cup whole-grain pasta
	steamed vegetables with olive oil
	sugar-free gelatin

Saturday menu

Breakfast	egg white, low-fat cheese, and vegetable omelet
	2 high-fiber whole-grain waffles
Snack	1 banana
Lunch	6 oz. broiled fish
	Steamed vegetables
	1 cup wild rice
Snack	1 cup plain nonfat Greek yogurt
Dinner	6 oz. steamed swordfish with capers and artichokes
	sautéed shrimp with garlic and olive oil
	1 cup whole-grain pasta
	sugar-free nonfat ice cream

Vegan Carbohydrate Rotation Menus

Monday menu

Breakfast	12 oz. nonfat soy milk (women) or nonfat rice milk (men) milk
	fresh fruit cocktail
Snack	1/2 cup unsalted nuts
Lunch	protein shake made with hemp protein isolate with almonds (men); soy protein isolate with almonds (women)
Snack	sugar-free iced tea
Dinner	steamed tofu with vegetables and low-sodium soy sauce
	sugar-free gelatin

Tuesday menu

Breakfast	protein shake made with hemp protein isolate with blackberries and cinnamon (men) soy protein isolate with black berries and cinnamon (women)
Snack	raw vegetables with low-sodium vegetable dip
Lunch	BBQ pepper, onion, corn 1 scoop protein powder with water red cabbage salad
Snack	1 fresh fruit of your choice
Dinner	wild rice mixed with black beans, lentils, and chopped vegetables fresh fruit cocktail

Wednesday menu

Breakfast	protein shake made with hemp protein isolate and banana (men) soy protein isolate and banana (women)
Snack	1 fresh fruit of your choice
Lunch	1 cup whole-grain pasta mixed with kidney beans, vegetables, and olive oil
Snack	sugar-free iced tea
Dinner	tofu stir-fried with mixed vegetables and olive oil sugar-free gelatin

Thursday menu

Breakfast	hemp protein powder shake (men); soy protein powder shake (women) wheat bran cereal with nonfat rice milk
Snack	1 fresh fruit of your choice

Lunch	brown rice mixed with lentils
	garden salad (greens, tomato, olives, olive oil, vinegar)
Snack	1 high-fiber English muffin
Dinner	tofu cooked in tomato sauce with spinach and sweet potato
	garden salad (greens, tomato, olives, olive oil, vinegar)
	1 cup fresh sliced pineapple

Friday menu

Breakfast	12 oz. nonfat rice milk (men) or soy milk (women)
	1 cup steel-cut oats with raisins
Snack	1 peach
Lunch	tofu, greens, olives, olive oil, vinegar
	whole-grain pita with hummus
Snack	sliced carrots and pickle
Dinner	wild rice mixed with lima beans and shredded tofu
	sautéed broccoli rabe (olive oil, garlic, red pepper)
	sugar-free gelatin

Saturday menu

Breakfast	smoothie with soy milk (women) or hemp milk (men) with protein isolate, blueberries, walnuts, 1/2 cup oats
Snack	apple slices and almonds
Lunch	whole-grain wrap with all-natural peanut butter
	zucchini salad
Snack	1 kiwi

Dinner   stir-fried tofu with red pepper, broccoli
sweet potato with olive oil

Inverted Cycle Carbohydrate Rotation Diet

By alternating your daily carbohydrate intake between low and high amounts, your body will be able to lose more of its body fat at a quicker rate. In the carbohydrate rotation diet, also called the inverted cycle diet, you begin the week eating the most carbs. You cut back a bit on the carbs each day after that for the rest of the week. On Sunday, you have a cheat day, where you eat as much of any foods you want, whenever you want. On Monday, you begin the rotation again. So, on Monday start the week with carbs at almost every meal. Over the course of the week, reduce your carbohydrate intake a bit each day by eating one less meal with carbs. On Saturday, have carbs at every meal. Sunday is your cheat day—enjoy it!

While you are on the inverted cycle diet, be sure to eat every 3 to 4 hours. You may have coffee and tea; use artificial sweetener. If you wish, you may have one glass of red or white wine with dinner. Drink plenty of water throughout the day: three to four quarts a day.

If you follow this approach, you will begin to feel very energized on Saturday and Sunday once you begin to ingest more carbohydrates.

By cycling and changing your diet's carbohydrate content on a daily basis, your metabolism varies as it adjusts to the different carbohydrates and calorie amounts of each meal. Each meal's portion size is well calculated for your body to digest it effectively. Most people eat portions that are too large. Whenever you eat too much food at one sitting, you will feel tired and lethargic because the body is overworking as it tries to digest all the food you've just piled into it. The extra food that it can't digest and use immediately will turn into fat.

After years of eating too much, you might develop type 2 diabetes. Eating meals with more carbohydrate calories than you need makes the body produce a lot of extra insulin, a hormone produced in your pancreas. After years of this, your body becomes less responsive to insulin.

To compensate, your body produces even more insulin to force your cells to respond. Eventually, the pancreas gets so overworked that it stops making enough insulin or even gives up completely. You develop type 2 diabetes and need to start taking a lot of drugs and even injecting insulin to keep your blood sugar under control.

Simply by following a diet that is lower in carbohydrates and higher in fiber will tremendously benefit your body. You'll stay lean and be much more likely to avoid diabetes and other health problems, such as high blood pressure and high cholesterol. A diet that is rich in healthy fats will keep your body running like a well-oiled machine. By continually alternating your body's carbohydrate intake, you will notice your physique looks leaner and your muscles feel firmer. By altering your carbohydrate intake daily or every few days, your body stays in fat-burning mode—it won't slow down its metabolism. The key to achieving maximum progress with your health and appearance is to constantly change your diet, workout times, and exercise routines. This will not give your body the chance to develop a pattern that stops weight loss and muscle growth. Constant change is the key to getting into the best shape ever!

Inverted Cycle Carbohydrate Rotation Diet

Monday menu: 5 meals, 4 with carbohydrates, 1 without

Breakfast	2 whole scrambled omega-3 eggs
	1 whole-grain bagel with all-natural peanut butter and fruit preserves
Snack	1 cup plain low-fat cottage cheese
Lunch	5 oz. sliced lean beef on whole-grain bread
	sliced pickle and cabbage salad
Snack	cucumber salad
Dinner	6 oz. baked turkey breast mixed with tomato, onion and sliced sweet potato

Greek salad with extra virgin olive oil
cantaloupe slices

Tuesday: 5 meals, 3 with carbohydrates, 2 without

Breakfast	1 cup egg whites, scrambled
	sugar-free toasted oats cereal with non fat soy milk (women) or nonfat milk (men)
Snack	1 fruit of your choice
Lunch	5 oz. grilled chicken breast with lemon and capers
	1 cup brown rice
	1 pickle
Snack	sliced cucumber and black olive salad with greens
Dinner	5 oz. lean pork with red peppers and olive oil
	1 cup whole-grain pasta with all-natural tomato sauce and extra virgin olive oil
	sliced kiwi

Wednesday: 5 meals, 2 with carbohydrates, 3 without

Breakfast	1 cup egg whites scrambled with spinach
	1 cup steel-cut oats mixed with fresh blueberries
Snack	1 nectarine
Lunch	6 oz. chicken breast with vegetables
	garden salad with extra virgin olive oil and almonds
Snack	steamed broccoli and cauliflower with low-sodium soy sauce

Dinner	6 oz. lean steak
	1 sweet potato
	broccoli rabe sautéed in extra virgin olive oil
	sugar-free gelatin

Thursday: 5 meals, 1 with carbohydrates, 4 without

Breakfast	2 soft-boiled omega-3 eggs
	2 sliced whole-grain bread
	wheat bran cereal with soy milk (women) or nonfat milk (men)
Snack	fresh fruit cocktail
Lunch	6 oz. turkey breast
	garden salad with extra virgin olive oil, vinegar, walnuts
Snack	1 sliced apple with cinnamon
Dinner	6 oz. chicken breast with lemon and black pepper
	steamed vegetables with extra virgin olive oil
	sugar-free gelatin

Friday: 5 meals, no carbohydrates

Breakfast	3 hard-boiled omega-3 eggs
	1 cup fresh blackberries
Snack	melon slices
Lunch	6 oz. grilled chicken breast with onion
	garden salad with extra virgin olive oil and vinegar
Snack	1 peach
Dinner	6 oz. BBQ lean steak
	BBQ mixed vegetables
	sugar-free gelatin

Saturday: 5 meals, all with carbohydrates

Breakfast	1 cup egg whites scrambled with tomato
	2 high-fiber pancakes with sugar-free syrup
Snack	1 banana, 1 slice rye bread
Lunch	5 oz. grilled lean steak
	sweet potato
Snack	1 cup fresh strawberries with heavy cream
Dinner	5 oz. turkey breast with extra virgin olive oil and capers
	1 cup wild rice
	garden salad with extra virgin olive oil and walnuts

Meatless Inverted Cycle Carbohydrate Rotation Diet

Monday menu: 5 meals, 4 with carbohydrates, 1 without

Breakfast	protein shake with soy (women) or whey (men) protein isolate, sliced pear, 6 walnuts, 1/2 cup steel-cut oats, water, ice
Snack	1 sliced apple with cinnamon
Lunch	shrimp sautéed with lemon and extra virgin olive oil
	1 cup wild rice
	cucumber salad
Snack	high-fiber whole-grain wrap with all-natural peanut butter
Dinner	broiled lobster tail with lemon and paprika
	baked sweet potato
	red cabbage salad
	sugar-free nonfat frozen yogurt

Tuesday: 5 meals, 3 with carbohydrates, 2 without

Breakfast	1 cup egg whites scrambled with spinach and tomato
	1 whole-grain bagel with fruit preserves
Snack	sliced banana with red grapes and walnuts
Lunch	5 oz. broiled salmon with extra virgin olive oil
	sautéed broccoli rabe
	1 cup brown rice
Snack	1 orange or grapefruit
Dinner	5 oz. BBQ fish with basil
	baked green or red pepper
	baked sweet potato
	sugar-free gelatin with fresh strawberries and sugar-free whipped cream

Wednesday: 5 meals, 2 with carbohydrates, 3 without

Breakfast	1 cup egg whites, scrambled with sliced red onion
	1/2 cup wheat bran mixed with fresh strawberries
Snack	1/2 cup unsalted mixed nuts
Lunch	Greek salad with octopus
Snack	melon slices
Dinner	6 oz. fried tilapia
	1 cup brown rice
	Brussels sprouts
	sugar-free vanilla pudding

Thursday: 5 meals, 1 with carbohydrates, 4 without

Breakfast	1 cup steel-cut oats mixed with 1 scoop soy (women) or whey (men) protein isolate, raisins
Snack	sliced kiwi and cherries
Lunch	sautéed shrimp with Asian vegetables
Snack	1 red grapefruit
Dinner	steamed clams with basil and extra virgin olive oil
	steamed lobster with lemon
	steamed peas
	corn on the cob
	sugar-free gelatin

Friday: 5 meals, none with carbohydrates

Breakfast	cup egg whites scrambled with spinach
	1 banana
Snack	1/2 cup unsalted mixed nuts
Lunch	1 can pink salmon
	garden salad
Snack	1 cup red grapes
Dinner	6 oz. grilled fish with parsley and capers
	steamed Brussels sprouts
	fresh fruit cocktail

Saturday: 5 meals, all with carbohydrates

Breakfast	1/3 cup cream of rice mixed with 1 scoop soy (women) or whey (men) protein isolate and 1 tablespoon all-natural peanut butter
Snack	1 hard-boiled omega-3 egg
	1 slice whole-grain bread

Lunch	1 can tuna in water with nonfat mayonnaise and chopped celery, served in a whole-grain wrap
Snack	12 oz. nonfat soy milk (women) or whole milk (men)
Dinner	5 oz. grilled fish with vegetables
	1 cup whole-grain pasta with extra virgin olive oil and all-natural tomato sauce
	fresh fruit cocktail with sugar-free whipped cream

Vegan Inverted Cycle Carbohydrate Rotation Diet

Monday: 5 meals, 4 with carbohydrates, 1 without

Breakfast	1 scoop soy (women) or whey (men) protein isolate mixed with water
	1/2 cup farina
Snack	1 sliced banana and walnuts
Lunch	1 cup brown rice
	1 cup lima beans
	garden salad
Snack	1 high-fiber English muffin with all-natural peanut butter
Dinner	stewed with all-natural tomato sauce mixed with steamed vegetables

Tuesday: 5 meals, 3 with carbohydrates, 2 without

Breakfast	1 glass nonfat soy milk (women) or rice milk (men)
	watermelon slices
Snack	2 slices whole-grain rye bread with all-natural peanut butter
Lunch	garden salad with beans

	1 cup whole-grain pasta with fresh tomato sauce
Snack	1 peach
Dinner	oven-baked tofu with tomato, broccoli, extra virgin olive oil, black pepper, sliced sweet potato
	sugar-free gelatin

Wednesday: 5 meals, 2 with carbohydrates, 3 without

Breakfast	1 cup high-fiber wheat bran cereal with nonfat soy milk (women), rice milk (men)
Snack	1 fresh fruit of your choice
Lunch	soy or rice milk shake with blueberries, water, ice
Snack	1/2 cup unsalted mixed nuts
Dinner	1 cup whole-grain pasta mixed with broccoli, red cabbage, lentils, extra virgin olive oil and garlic
	1 sliced pear with cherries

Thursday: 5 meals, 1 with carbohydrates, 4 without

Breakfast	2/3 cup oat bran mixed with soy or rice milk, cinnamon
	1 cup red grapes
Lunch	tofu salad with greens, extra virgin olive oil, vinegar
Snack	1 cup cherries
Dinner	lentil soup with tofu and red pepper garden salad with almonds, extra virgin olive oil, vinegar
	1 peach

Friday: 5 meals, none with carbohydrates

Breakfast	protein shake with 1 scoop soy protein isolate, 6 almonds, 1 small apple, water, ice
Snack	1 cup raisins
Lunch	tofu with steamed vegetables
Snack	1 cup raspberries
Dinner	oven-baked tofu with onion, tomato, garlic
	garden salad with extra virgin olive oil
	sliced fresh pineapple

Saturday: 5 meals, all with carbohydrates

Breakfast	1 glass soy milk (women) or rice milk (men)
	1/2 cup steel cut oats
Snack	1 apple, 1 tablespoon all-natural peanut butter
Lunch	1 cup whole-grain pasta mixed with olive oil and beans
	garden salad with extra virgin olive oil
Snack	1 grapefruit, 10 walnuts
Dinner	1 cup brown rice
	tofu salad with extra virgin olive oil
	sliced fresh pineapple

Increasing Carbohydrate Rotation Diet

This particular approach differs from the other carbohydrate rotation diets because you begin the week consuming few carbohydrates and increase the amount by one carbohydrate meal each day as the week progresses. Sunday, of course, is the cheat day, where you may eat whatever and whenever you desire. Cheat days are very important to have once a week because they give you a mental break. Feeling free to cheat and eat whatever you want reduces the stress of dieting. You're much more able to stick with the meal plan for long enough to achieve real success.

Always be sure to drink plenty of plain water every day. I recommend three to four quarts (8 to 12 glasses) daily. You can also drink coffee, tea, herbal tea, and iced tea. Avoid adding milk or sugar to these. Also avoid drinks with added sugar, such as soda, energy drinks, fruit juices, and similar beverages. Artificially sweetened drinks in limited amounts are acceptable. You can have one glass of red or white wine with dinner if you wish. Wine is optional, however—skip it if you don't like it or don't want the effects of alcohol.

Carb rotation diets constantly "trick" the body by feeding it different carbohydrate amounts each day and switching on the body's own fat-burning mechanism. Carb rotation diets are a popular fat-loss method with competitive bodybuilders, because they know how well they work. The body is very resilient and will adjust itself to any sort of workout routine and diet. If you follow the same approach every day, your body will eventually get used to them and you will stop seeing improvement. To avoid this, and also to keep things interesting for you, it's best to make constant changes by continually alternating meal plans and exercise regimens. This will cause your body to burn more fat, because it is constantly changing its metabolism in an attempt to adjust to the different carbohydrate amounts. The key to a successful diet is to keep your body "confused" by constantly alternating your food intake.

In this variation of carbohydrate rotation, you increase your carbohydrate intake each day as the week progresses. By the end of the week, your skin will feel tight, your muscles will feel solid, and you will have more overall energy.

Increasing Carbohydrate Rotation Diet
Monday: 5 meals, no carbohydrates
Breakfast   2 hard-boiled omega-3 eggs
                                  1 cup fresh strawberries

Snack	10 unsalted walnuts
Lunch	6 oz. broiled chicken breast
	garden salad
Snack	1 cup raisins
Dinner	6 oz. broiled lean steak
	mixed steamed vegetables with olive oil
	watermelon slices

Tuesday: 5 meals, 1 with carbohydrates, 4 without

Breakfast	1 cup egg whites scrambled with tomato omelet
	1/2 cup farina
Snack	1 red grapefruit
Lunch	6 oz. turkey breast
	Brussels sprouts
Snack	1 plum
Dinner	6 oz. grilled London broil
	mixed vegetables
	sugar-free gelatin

Wednesday: 5 meals, 2 with carbohydrates, 3 without

Breakfast	1 cup sugar-free oats cereal with almonds and 1 scoop soy (women) or whey (men) protein isolate with nonfat soy milk (women) or nonfat milk (men)
Snack	1 whole-grain bagel with all-natural peanut butter and fruit preserves
Lunch	5 oz. grilled lean chopped meat mixed with onion
	heart of palm salad with extra virgin olive oil
Snack	1 cup cherries

Dinner	6 oz. lean pork with olive oil, carrots, broccoli, asparagus and olive salad
	fresh fruit cocktail

Thursday: 5 meals, 3 with carbohydrates, 2 without

Breakfast	1 cup egg whites scrambled with spinach
	1/2 cup quinoa with 8 walnuts
Snack	1 cup raspberries
Lunch	5 oz. turkey breast with lettuce, tomato and whole-wheat pita
Snack	1 banana
Dinner	5 oz. grilled lamb chop
	baked sweet potato
	avocado salad

Friday: 5 meals, 4 with carbohydrates, 1 without

Breakfast	2 pancakes made with 1 scoop whey (men) or soy (women) protein isolate combined with high-fiber fiber pancake mix
Snack	1 cup plain nonfat Greek yogurt
Lunch	6 oz. lean hamburger with tomato, pickle on whole-grain bun
Snack	1 sliced mango
Dinner	5 oz. sautéed London broil with mushrooms and olive oil
	Greek salad
	1 cup wild rice
	sugar-free gelatin with strawberries and sugar-free whipped cream

Saturday: 5 meals, all with carbohydrates

Breakfast	2 soft-boiled omega-3 eggs whole-grain high-fiber wrap
Snack	1 cup plain low-fat cottage cheese
Lunch	5 oz. chicken breast with lettuce and tomato on 7-grain bread
Snack	1 pumpernickel bagel with fruit preserves
Dinner	5 oz. turkey breast with olive oil, carrots and onion 1 cup whole-grain pasta mixed with sautéed spinach and extra virgin olive oil papaya fruit cocktail

Meatless Increasing Carbohydrate Rotation Diet

Monday: 5 meals, no carbohydrates

Breakfast	1 cup egg whites, scrambled watermelon slices
Snack	1 pickle
Lunch	6 oz. steamed salmon with mixed vegetables
Snack	1 red grapefruit
Dinner	6 oz. broiled fish red cabbage and beets salad

Tuesday: 5 meals, 1 with carbohydrates, 4 without

Breakfast	2 soft-boiled omega-3 eggs with a toasted whole-wheat bagel
Snack	1 cup red grapes
Lunch	6 oz. grilled fish with lemon and capers green beans with olive oil
Snack	1 red grapefruit

Dinner	6 oz. grilled white fish with garlic and lemon
	steamed kale
	corn on the cob
	sugar-free gelatin

Wednesday: 5 meals, 2 with carbohydrates, 3 without

Breakfast	protein shake made with 1 scoop soy (women) or whey (men) protein isolate mixed with 8 almonds, 1 banana, water, ice
Snack	1/2 cup unsalted peanuts
Lunch	baked tofu with steamed vegetables
	tomato and cucumber salad with olive oil
Snack	fresh fruit cocktail
Dinner	6 oz. grilled salmon with black pepper and lime
	1 cup brown rice
	salad with onion and beets, extra virgin olive oil
	1 kiwi

Thursday: 5 meals, 3 with carbohydrates, 2 without

Breakfast	1 cup steel-cut oats with 2 tablespoons all-natural peanut butter
Snack	1 cup plain nonfat Greek yogurt with 8 unsalted almonds
Lunch	octopus salad with olives
	toasted whole-grain pita with 2 tablespoons hummus
Snack	1 apple

Dinner	shrimp sautéed with olive oil, red pepper, and garlic
	1 cup brown rice
	heart of palm salad
	1 nectarine

Friday: 5 meals, 4 with carbohydrates, 1 without

Breakfast	1 cup egg whites scrambled with tomato and red pepper
	sugar-free wheat bran cereal with soy milk (women) or nonfat milk (men)
Snack	1 toasted whole-wheat bagel with all-natural peanut butter and fruit preserves
Lunch	steamed shrimp with vegetables
	1 cup brown rice
Snack	1 orange
Dinner	steamed lobster with lemon
	baked sweet potato
	cucumber, tomato, and olive salad
	1 kiwi

Saturday: 5 meals, all with carbohydrates

Breakfast	1 glass soy milk (women) or nonfat milk (men)
	1/2 cup plain oat bran with 6 unsalted walnuts
Snack	1 low-fat protein bar
Lunch	tuna in water with chopped celery and onion
	whole-grain wrap
	1 cup cherries
Snack	plain low-fat cottage cheese with sliced pineapple

Dinner	broiled octopus with extra virgin olive oil and paprika
	1 cup whole-grain pasta
	garden salad with unsalted mixed nuts, extra virgin olive oil and vinegar
	nonfat sugar-free frozen yogurt topped with 6 unsalted almonds

Vegan Increasing Carbohydrate Rotation Diet

Monday: 5 meals, no carbohydrates

Breakfast	protein shake made with 1 scoop soy (women) or hemp (men) protein isolate blended with 1 cup strawberries, water, ice
Snack	1 tablespoon almond butter
Lunch	lentil and tofu soup with vegetables
	garden salad with 10 cashews, olive oil, vinegar
Snack	1 pomegranate
Dinner	stir-fried tofu with mushrooms and olive oil
	steamed cabbage with spicy mustard
	sugar-free frozen ice pop

Tuesday: 5 meals, 1 with carbohydrates, 4 without

Breakfast	1 glass soy milk (women) or rice milk (men)
	1 cup cream of rice with 8 unsalted cashews
Snack	raw carrots with vegetable dip
Lunch	tofu, mixed greens, red pepper, extra virgin olive oil and vinegar
Snack	1 cup unsweetened coconut pieces

Dinner — tofu with steamed broccoli and garlic
avocado salad
kiwi mixed with strawberries

Wednesday: 5 meals, 2 with carbohydrates, 3 without

Breakfast	1 cup steel-cut oats mixed with all-natural peanut butter
Snack	1 papaya
Lunch	1 cup whole-grain pasta mixed with tofu and all-natural tomato sauce
Snack	1 mango
Dinner	1 cup wild rice mixed with red beans and red pepper
	avocado and cucumber salad with extra virgin olive oil and vinegar
	1 apple

Thursday: 5 meals, 3 with carbohydrates, 2 without

Breakfast	1 cup sugar-free toasted oats cereal with soy milk (women) or rice milk (men) mixed with 8 unsalted cashews
Snack	1 banana
Lunch	baked beans
	1 cup brown rice
	avocado salad
Snack	1 pomegranate
Dinner	tofu with stewed tomatoes, with basil, red pepper
	vegetable soup
	1 cup sliced strawberries with cinnamon and nonfat rice milk

Friday: 5 meals, 4 with carbohydrates, 1 without

Breakfast	protein shake with 1 scoop soy (women) or hemp (men) protein isolate blended with 1/2 cup oats, 1/2 cup blueberries, 6 unsalted walnuts, water, ice
Snack	high-fiber English muffin with all-natural peanut butter
Lunch	tofu with greens, tomato, olives, vinegar, and extra virgin olive oil
Snack	1 Asian pear
Dinner	1 cup wild rice mixed with chopped Brussels sprouts
	lentil soup
	corn on the cob and red pepper
	pineapple slices

Saturday: 5 meals, all with carbohydrates

Breakfast	1 cup steel-cut oats mixed with 1 scoop soy (women) or hemp (men) protein isolate, sliced banana
Snack	1 whole-grain wrap with all-natural almond butter
Lunch	1 cup brown rice mixed with lentils
	sliced cucumbers
Dinner	tofu stir-fried with onion and mushrooms
	heart of palm salad with vinegar and extra-virgin olive oil
	1 cup strawberries with rice milk

Which Diet Fits You Best?

The secret to an effective diet is choosing the one that you like best. You must accept and understand that getting into great shape is not an overnight procedure but rather a long-term commitment. I'm sure you've seen many weight-loss advertisements that promise "lose weight fast." These companies make these statements strictly to gain your business. There is no such thing as "lose weight fast" when it comes to creating a healthy and attractive body. Rushing into a restrictive, low-calorie diet in order to lose weight quickly will literally wreak havoc on your body. The faster the body sheds its fat, the worse it will look. Lean muscle tissue will be consumed in the process of basically starving yourself and your metabolism will slow down. And that's not to mention possible dehydration and other health hazards—even a heart attack—that could be caused by such rapid weight loss.

For safe and effective weight loss, the body should only shed one to two pounds per week. Once you begin to lose more than that, you will begin to lose water and lean muscle tissue, something that you never want. By gradually reducing your caloric intake, your body will slowly and safely tap into its own stored energy source (your body fat) for fuel. This slow and continual transition will cause you to burn excess fat at a safe and healthy pace. You may believe that losing only one to two pounds a week isn't enough. It is when you multiply one to two pounds a week by several months. You could lose between 10 and 20 pounds in just a few months if you're consistent about sticking to your diet. Remember that you're not on a weight-loss diet, you're on life-improving lifestyle diet. This diet is the one you'll be able to stick with, especially once you've "tasted" the results.

Losing two pounds per week of body fat will amount to losing a lot over time. However, after several months, your rate of weight loss will slow down as your body adjusts itself to your lower caloric intake by lowering its metabolism. That's why it's helpful to "trick" your body by alternating your diet. By alternating your carbohydrate intake with a carb rotation meal plan, you "confuse" your body. It won't be able to adjust your metabolism downward as easily, so you'll experience better results and lose more fat. The constant changing of the diet renders the best results.

When people begin a diet they tend to see relatively quick results early on. After several weeks or months, however, they seem to hit a plateau where weight loss stalls. They decide the diet no longer works and they quit. This is a common mistake. All too often, people who get frustrated by their diet regain all the weight they lost. To avoid plateaus and frustration, I stress the principle of constant change, continually alternating all aspects of your diet.

Constant change will help you other ways as well. You'll stay more interested in your diet and won't get bored as you normally would if you were to consume the same foods all the time. Having variety in your weight-loss program will facilitate the entire process of getting into shape. I have been on many different diets over the years and the most important thing I've learned is that it is very important always to eat different foods.

The combination of frequently alternating the foods you enjoy eating and experiencing steady results by feeling and looking better is the greatest motivation of all! As you start to look and feel better all the time, you will become extremely excited about maintaining this new and better lifestyle. Getting into shape and developing the body of your dreams will no longer seem like a chore, but rather, an exciting adventure!

Chapter 12
Sculpting Your Body

We're now ready to begin Phase IV, fitness. Before beginning this phase, let's look back at the three previous phases.

Phase I: Motivation. This is where it all begins. You have made the conscious decision to improve the way you look and feel. You no longer want to feel sluggish, not be proud of the way your body appears, and no longer miss out on life simply because you wished you were in better shape. Phase I involves changing your mindset and making the decision to change your body and health for the better.

Phase II: Sleep. During this phase, the importance of having adequate sleep is stressed. Before you are ready to begin the next phase of dieting, you need to make sure you understand the importance of giving your body enough sleep and rest time. If you don't make Phase II part of your life, you won't be able to effectively move on to the next. Allow yourself plenty of sleep and rest time. Seven to nine hours of sleep should be enough to prepare your body for a successful health and fitness program.

Phase III: Diet. In this phase, you begin to incorporate the meal plans that are key to weight loss and getting into shape.

Phase IV: Exercise. If you've followed all the previous phases, your body is now ready to begin an exercise program that will sculpt your body. You will begin to use resistance (weight) and cardiovascular training. Weight training will tone and strengthen your body; cardiovascular exercises will increase your endurance and strengthen your heart. During this phase. you will begin noticing vast improvements in strength and tone. Your body will noticeably begin to sculpt itself into that of an attractive and healthy individual, while you will look and feel years younger.

Exercising is an integral part of creating an attractive and healthy physique. There are many ways to exercise, but they all come down to two aspects: aerobic and anaerobic. . Aerobic training gets your heart rate up through cardiovascular activity such as jogging, running, swimming, biking, calisthenics, and using exercise machines such as treadmills and elliptical. Sports are a great and fun way to get aerobic exercise. Aerobic training involves non-resistant exercising, which means the exercises don't include weight-training (resistance) or any other muscle-building workouts.

Cardiovascular workouts develop and strengthen the heart muscle and improve the body's blood circulation. Having a stronger heart is extremely important for longevity and quality of life. When your heart beats strongly and your have good circulation, your body operates more efficiently, with much more energy and drive—including increased libido and cognitive brain function. When you are in good cardiovascular shape, you will definitely feel the difference. You will feel as if you have more jump in your step!

Anaerobic training is exercising the body's muscles in order to increase their strength and mass. This is done mostly through resistance training, also called weight training. Anaerobic exercise has many benefits for the body other than improving its appearance by building muscle. Although muscles always seem to be the primary reason most people have starting weight training, they soon find other benefits. This type of exercise increases bone mass and strength as well. As we age, we all slowly lose bone mass and density. For some people, the loss is so great over time that they develop osteoporosis, bones that are weak, brittle, and break easily. Resistance training also strengthens ligaments and tendons, preventing them from wearing down and causing joint injuries. If you have arthritis in a joint, strengthening the muscles, ligaments, and tendons can help stabilize the joint and may help it be less painful.

Resistance training also has a positive effect on the body's hormones. Anaerobic exercise increases testosterone levels in men. In everyone, it decreases levels of the stress hormone cortisol level. If you have blood sugar issues or type 2 diabetes, anaerobic exercise (and also aerobic exercise) improve insulin resistance and lower your blood sugar.

When a man's natural levels of testosterone are high and his cortisol levels are low, he will be able to develop lean muscle tissue and lose fat most efficiently. Lifting weights and any other type of resistance exercising will strengthen your entire body and give you a more toned and sculpted look. You will also be able to shed unwanted body fat at a quicker pace while actually being able to burn more calories. This may seem hard to believe, but it's true. Resistance training builds muscle tissue—and the larger your muscles, the more calories they burn even if you're just sitting still.

Think of shopping for a car that has two different engine options: a small six cylinder or large V8. The larger motor has more power than the smaller one, but it also consumes more fuel. The same applies to the body: the larger the muscles, the stronger you are and the more food the body will need to feed the larger muscles. Just like the car with the more powerful motor, it uses more fuel whether it is driving at 10 or 60 miles per hour. The same applies to your body. Regardless of your activity level, the larger, stronger muscles will always require more calories to sustain them. The more resistance training you do, the more food you will be able to eat without gaining body fat. Resistance training has no negative drawbacks—it's why I recommend it to everyone.

<a>Resistance Training Exercises

Resistance training workouts can be approached in different ways. Some people prefer to train different body parts on different days: legs on one day, upper body on the next, abdomen after that, for instance. Within a week's time, all of the body's major muscle groups have been exercised at least once. Others prefer to train the whole body a few times a week. Which approach works best? They all do, at different levels of your training. "Shocking" the body by constantly alternating the training regimen, usually by increasing and decreasing the number of times per week, has been proven to work very effectively. It's a good way to break through the plateaus and stagnation points that often occur during training. Changing your workout regimen will also allow you to increase the fun factor, which means you won't get bored while exercising.

Weight lifting is the most popular form of resistance training, but it's not for everybody. If you don't enjoy it, you can try an alternative form. Calisthenics, for instance, is a form of training that involves using your own body weight as the resistance. You're probably familiar with calisthenics exercises such as push-ups and pull-ups. These exercises use the arms to lift the weight of the body.

Many people think the best way to develop strength and lean muscle tissue is by weight training, but this isn't really true. For example, have you ever watched a top-level gymnastics event such as the Olympics? If you have, then I'm sure you noticed the strength and muscular development of the gymnasts. These athletes are typically very lean and muscular. Their physiques were developed by calisthenics—lifting their own body weight. Your body will achieve its best results by combining both weight training and calisthenics exercises throughout your entire resistance training regimen.

The Major Muscle Groups
Upper Body (pushing)
Chest
Front deltoid (shoulder)
Triceps

Upper Body (pulling)
Back
Rear deltoid (shoulder)
Biceps

Lower Body (pushing)
Gluteus maximus (buttocks)
Quadriceps (thigh)
Rear calves

Lower Body (pulling)
Hamstrings (thigh)
Front calves

Core (stabilizing)
Abdominals
Lower back
Intercostals (rib cage area)
Serratus (shoulder blade and back area)
Neck

For every physical movement your body does, muscles are either pulling or pushing—even both in some motions. Regardless of which muscle group is being trained, you must allow adequate time to heal from the tiny muscle tears that occur after every workout. The tears are perfectly normal—they're how you build muscles.

Muscles strengthen and increase in size in a two-step process: first, breaking down and second, healing. The breaking down occurs during training. During resistance training, the strain on the muscle causes very small tears. In other words, lifting weights breaks down the muscle tissue. The second phase is how the body repairs the torn muscle tissue. Your body needs two things for the repair process: protein from your diet and rest time for the repair to happen. During each repair period, the muscle becomes larger and stronger. You need to allow at least 48 hours of rest time after a workout for the muscles to completely heal themselves. For example, if you were to train biceps on Monday it would be best to wait until at least Wednesday to train them again. On Tuesday you could train another body part while allowing the biceps to heal.

For muscles to grow, they must be broken down through resistance training and repaired by way of proper nutrition, rest, and sleep. Frequently alternating your entire fitness program by changing the workouts and meal plans will keep your body from becoming too accustomed to the program. If all you do is repeat the same routines, your progress will eventually slow and then cease. Always "shocking" the body by changing up your exercise routine will lead to better results—and it will keep you from getting into a boring fitness rut.

If you're new to resistance training, I very strongly suggest that you join a well-equipped gym and work with an experienced trainer to learn how to do the exercises safely and with good form. This is crucial to avoiding injury and getting the most from your workout. I also suggest watching free videos online to see the right way to do the exercises and get ideas for ways to vary your routine. YouTube has thousands of these; another good source is boydbuilding.com.

Older adults should be especially careful to use good form to avoid injury. Start slowly, with light weights, and gradually build up to the weights that give you a challenging workout without straining you.

Muscle Groups and Their Exercises

Chest	*Back*	*Legs*
flat barbell bench press	pull-ups	leg extensions
inclined barbell bench press	chin-ups	leg curls
decline barbell bench press	lat machine pull-downs	leg presses
flat dumbbell bench press	seated row	lunges
incline dumbbell bench press	barbell row	squats
incline decline press	T-bar row	stiff-legdeadlifts
push-ups	dumbbell row	sissy squats
pull-ups	hyper-extensions	front squats
dumbbell flyes	back squats	standing calf raises
pec-dec	Smith machine	squats
dip	Smith machine	front squats
cable crossovers	Smith machine	stiff leg deadlifts

Shoulders
front barbell shoulder press
dumbbell lateral raises
behind-the-neck shoulder press
dumbbell bent-over lateral raises
front dumbbell press
front barbell raises
behind-the-neck dumbbell press
front dumbbell raises
barbell upright row
Smith machine front shoulder press
dumbbell upright row
Smith machine behind-the-neck press
cable lateral raises
cable bent-over lateral raises

Biceps/Triceps
standing barbell curl
lying triceps extension
standing dumbbell curl
seated triceps extension
preacher curl
dumbbell kickback
dumbbell hammer curl
close-grip barbell bench press
cable curl
cable push-down
cable preacher curl
inverted cable push-down
seated dumbbell curl
seated overhead dumbbell triceps extension
dumbbell concentration curl
dips

reverse dips

Calves/Forearms
seated calf raises
standing calf raises
donkey calf raises
upside-down calf raises
wrist curls
inverted wrist curls

Neck/Abdominals
front neck bridges
rear neck bridges
sit-ups
crunches
inverted crunches
leg raises
hanging leg raises

Trapezius/Shoulder
barbell shrugs
dumbbell shrugs
close-grip upright rows

Exercise Routines

When training, the object is to exercise each muscle group at least one time per week. Remember, each muscle needs at least 48 hours to heal itself after it has been trained. This means your can exercise your entire body as often as three times per week, because you this will allow at least 48 hours between training the same body part.

You may train each body part once, twice, or three times per week. For example, you may exercise your leg muscles either every Wednesday if you want to train them once per week; every Monday and Thursday or Tuesday and Friday, if you are training them twice per week;

every Monday, Wednesday, and Friday, if you are training them three times per week. Regardless of the days of the week that you choose to exercise, you must rest that particular muscle at least one day in between workouts.

The most popular regimen for weight training is exercising each major muscle group once per week. I, on the other hand, often alternate my workouts, training each body part either once, twice, or three times per week. This method keeps the body in "constant confusion" by never allowing it to become immune to the same workouts and limit its progress. Changing the workouts on a frequent basis has proven to render the best results.

Weekly Full Body Training

A muscle grows in strength and mass when it is both exercised through resistance and allowed to heal immediately following. The amount of healing time needed is usually at least 48 hours. For this reason, people tend to take at least one day off between workouts. Training the entire body across a week, using a five-day exercise schedule, seems to be the most popular method. Many of the top professional athletes train this way. Giving the body an entire week to heal itself will enable you to exercise each particular muscle group with extreme intensity, knowing that adequate rest will follow. This training method is called "muscle prioritization," because you exercise only one muscle group each day—that particular muscle group is prioritized. I have used this method many times and have always appreciated the shorter and more intense workouts, followed by the long rest time to allow my muscles to heal.

I am a firm believer in changing the workout regimen once your progress comes to a plateau. Incorporating muscle prioritization can be very beneficial toward achieving your fitness goal.

Resistance Exercise Workouts

If you choose to follow the muscle prioritization approach, you will be working out five days a week. You will train a different muscle group each day. By the end of the five days, all your muscles will have been trained. Start any day of the week you want, as long as you continue for five days straight and then take two days off in a row.

If you can't get to the gym five days in a row, no worries—you can still get a great, full-body workout in less time. In fact, you can even do just one workout a week and exercise every muscle. I show you exactly how in the section below. Follow the exercise recommendations and schedule closely to make sure you exercise all the main muscle groups. For the best results, it's also important to rest on the designated days. On those days, you should still be active. Have some fun—ride your bike, go for a walk or a run, play a sport, go dancing. You'll soon notice that resistance exercise is not only giving your muscles more tone and definition, it's increasing your energy level and endurance. You also now have more power—the combination of speed and strength.

If you're new to resistance training, a rep (short for repetition) is one complete motion of the exercise. A set is a specific number of reps, usually ten or twelve. Give yourself a few minutes to rest between sets. However, sometime supersetting—doing the sets without resting in between and moving on to the next exercise without resting—can be a fun challenge.

Start with very light weights, but make them heavy enough so that the last few reps of each set are hard, but not too hard. If they're too difficult, reduce the amount of weight until you find the number that's right. If the exercise is too easy, increase the weight—don't just do more reps or sets. Likewise, if the exercise is too hard, decrease the weight—don't decrease the number of reps or sets.

Once again, I strongly urge you to find a gym that's convenient for you and has an experienced trainer who can teach you how to use the weights and machines safely and correctly. This will help you avoid injury, boredom, and frustration and get you to good results a lot faster.

Many of the older adults I work with have some health issues, such as arthritis and diabetes. In most cases, a health problem isn't a reason to avoid physical activity. In fact, diabetes, arthritis, and even heart problems are usually helped by exercise. Before you begin a weight-training program, however, you *must* check with your doctor to make sure it's safe for you. Your doctor may suggest some limits to your exercise, especially when you first begin working out. Be sure to keep these in mind at all times; also be sure to tell your trainer about them. A good trainer can suggest exercises that will work around any limitations you may have.

Any amount of exercise is better than no exercise—do what you can and don't be afraid to push yourself a little.

Training Schedules for Beginners
Five Days a Week

	Sets	Repetitions
Day 1: Chest		
Flat barbell bench press	3	12
Incline barbell bench press	3	12
Day 2: Back		
Lat machine pull-down	3	12
Seated cable row	3	12
Day 3: Shoulders		
Lateral dumbbell raise	2	12
Upright barbell row	2	12
Front barbell press	2	12
Day 4: Biceps, triceps, abs		
Standing dumbbell curl	2	12
Seated preacher curl	2	12
Cable push-down	3	12
Inverted grip cable push-down	3	12
Sit-ups	2	20

Day 5: Legs, calves
Leg extension	2	12
Leg curl	2	12
Lunges	2	12
Seated calf raise	2	12

Day 6: Rest day
Day 7: Rest day

Four Days a Week

	Sets	Repetitions
Day 1: Chest, triceps		
Flat barbell bench press	3	12
Triceps cable push-down	3	12
Incline barbell bench press	3	12
Inverted grip cable push-down	3	12
Day 2: Back, Biceps, Abs		
Lat machine pull-down	3	12
Standing dumbbell curl	3	12
Seated cable row	3	12
Seated preacher curl	3	12
Sit-ups	2	20

Day 3: Rest day

Day 4: Shoulders, abs		
Lateral dumbbell raises	2	12
Upright barbell row	2	12
Front barbell press	2	12
Leg raises	2	10
Day 5: Legs, calves		
Leg extension	2	12

Leg curl	2	12
Lunges	2	12
Seated calf raise	2	12

Day 6: Rest day
Day 7: Rest day

Three Days a Week

	Sets	Repetitions
Day 1: Chest, back, abs		
Flat barbell bench press	3	12
Lat machine pull-down	3	12
Incline barbell bench press	3	12
Seated cable row	3	12
Sit-ups	1	20

Day 2: Rest day

Day 3: Shoulders, Triceps, Biceps, Abs		
Lateral dumbbell raises	2	12
Upright barbell row	2	12
Front barbell press	2	12
Triceps cable push-down	3	12
Inverted grip cable push-down	3	12
Standing dumbbell curl	3	12
Seated preacher curl	3	12
Crunches	1	20

Day 4: Rest day

Day 5: Legs, calves		
Leg extension	2	12
Leg curl	2	12

	Sets	Repetitions
Lunges	2	12
Seated calf raise	2	12

Day 6: Rest day
Day 7: Rest day

Two Days a Week

	Sets	Repetitions
Day 1: Upper body		
Flat barbell bench press	3	12
Incline barbell bench press	3	10
Triceps cable push-down	2	15
Seated trips extension	2	12
Wide grip lat machine pull-down	3	8
Seated cable row	3	10
Seated preacher curl	2	12
Standing dumbbell curl	2	10
Lateral dumbbell raises	2	12
Upright row	2	12
Machine shoulder press	2	10
Day 2: Lower body		
Leg extension	3	15
Leg curl	3	12
Lunges	3	10
Leg press	3	10
Stiff leg dead-lift	3	10
Seated calf raise	3	15
Sit-ups	5	10

Note: Choose any two days; they do not have to be consecutive

One Day a Week

	Sets	Repetitions
Flat barbell bench press	2	10
Incline barbell bench press	2	10
Pec-dec machine	2	12
Wide grip lat machine pull-down	2	10
Close grip lat machine pull-down	2	10
Seated cable row	2	10
Machine shoulder press	2	10
Upright row	2	10
Lateral dumbbell raises	2	12
Standing barbell curl	2	10
Seated dumbbell curl	2	10
Triceps cable push-down	2	15
Lying triceps extension	2	10
Crunches	5	10
Leg extension	2	15
Leg curl	2	15
Lunges	2	10
Hack squats	2	12
Seated calf raise	3	15

Training Schedules for Intermediates

Five Days a Week

Day 1: Chest, cardio, abs
stationary bicycle, treadmill, or elliptical machine: 30 minutes

	Sets	Repetitions
Flat barbell bench press	3	10
Incline barbell bench press	3	10
Cable cross-overs	3	15
Sit-ups	2	15

Day 2: Back, cardio
Close grip lat machine pull-down	3	10
Wide grip lat machine pull-down	3	10
Seated cable row	3	10

Brisk walk: 20 minutes

Day 3: Shoulders, traps, abs
Front barbell shoulder press	3	10
Wide grip upright barbell row	3	10
Lateral dumbbell raises	3	10
Barbell shrugs	3	10
Crunches	2	15

Day 4: Biceps, triceps
Triceps cable push-down	3	10
Close grip barbell bench press	3	10
Inverted grip triceps cable push-downs	2	10
Standing barbell curl	3	10
Seated dumbbell curl	3	10
Preacher curl	2	10

Light jog: 15 minutes

Day 5: Legs, calves, abs
Leg extension	3	10
Leg curl	3	10
Lunges	3	10
Leg press	3	10
Leg raises	2	10

Day 6: Rest day
Day 7: Rest day

Four Days a Week
Day 1: Chest, triceps, abs, cardio

	Sets	Repetitions
Flat bench dumbbell flyes	2	10
Incline barbell bench press	3	10
Flat barbell bench press	3	10
Triceps cable push-down	3	10
Lying triceps extension	3	10
Close grip barbell bench press	2	10
Inverted crunches	2	20

Elliptical machine: 30 minutes

Day 2: Back, biceps, abs, cardio

	Sets	Repetitions
Close grip lat machine pull-down	3	10
Wide grip lat machine pull-down	3	10
Seated cable row	3	10
Dumbbell concentration curl	3	10
Standing barbell curl	3	10
Cable curl	2	10
Crunches	2	20

Stationary bicycle: 30 minutes

Day 3: Rest day

Day 4: Shoulders, abs, traps, cardio
Brisk walk: 30 minutes

	Sets	Repetitions
Machine shoulder press	3	10
Cable lateral raises	3	10
Rear delt machine exercise	3	10
Close grip upright barbell row	3	10
Sit-ups	2	20

Day 5: Legs, calves, abs, cardio
Treadmill: 30 minutes

Leg extension	3	10
Leg press	3	10
Leg curl	3	10
Lunges	3	10
Leg raises	2	20

Day 6: Rest day
Day 7: Rest day

Three Days a Week
Day 1: Chest, biceps, triceps, abs, cardio

	Sets	Repetitions
Incline bench dumbbell flyes	3	10
Incline barbell bench press	3	10
Push-ups	3	10
Standing cable curl	3	15
Preacher curl machine	3	12
Dumbbell concentration curls	2	10
Lying triceps extension	3	10
Dumbbell triceps kick-back	3	15
Cable triceps push-down	2	12
Sit-ups	2	20

Light jog: 30 minutes

Day 2: Rest day

Day 3: Back, shoulders, traps, abs, cardio

	Sets	Repetitions
Wide grip lat machine pull-down	3	10
Close grip lat machine pull-down	3	10
Seated cable row	3	10

	Sets	Repetitions
Machine shoulder press	3	10
Dumbbell lateral raises	3	12
Bent over dumbbell lateral raises	3	12
Dumbbell shrugs	3	10
Crunches	2	20

Stationary bicycle: 30 minutes

Day 4: Rest day

Day 5: Legs, calves, abs, cardio

	Sets	Repetitions
Leg extension	3	15
Leg curl	3	15
Lunges	3	10
Hack squats	3	10
Standing calf raise	2	20
Leg raises	2	20

Elliptical machine: 30 minutes

Two Days a Week
Day 1: Upper body, cardio

	Sets	Repetitions
Wide grip lat machine pull-down	3	12
Seated cable row	3	12
Pull-ups	2	8
Cable lateral raises	3	12
Front barbell shoulder press	3	10
Bent-over cable lateral raises	2	12
Close grip upright row	2	10
Standing barbell curl	5	10
Lying triceps extension	5	10
Incline barbell press	5	12
Decline barbell press	4	12

	Sets	Repetitions
Crunches	2	20

Stationary bicycle: 30 minutes

Day 2: Lower body, cardio

	Sets	Repetitions
Treadmill: 30 minutes		
Leg extension	3	15
Leg curl	3	15
Lunges	3	12
Front squats	3	10
Stiff-leg dead lift	3	10
Seated calf raise	2	20
Sit-ups	5	10

Note: Each workout should be completed within 60 to 90 minutes. Choose any two days; they do not have to be consecutive

One Day a Week

	Sets	Repetitions
Elliptical machine: 30 minutes		
Leg extension	3	12
Leg curl	3	12
Lunges	3	10
Hack squats	2	10
Stiff-leg dead lift	2	10
Incline barbell press	4	10
Flat bench dumbbell press	4	10
T-bar row	4	10
Pull-ups	4	8
Concentration curl	4	15
Seated triceps extension	4	12
Upright row	4	10
Front barbell shoulder press	4	8
Standing calf raises	3	20

Leg raises   4   12

Note: The entire workout should be completed within 75 to 90 minutes.

Advanced Resistance Exercise Training Schedule
Five Days a Week

	Sets	Repetitions
Day 1: Chest, cardio, abs		
Outside run: 30 minutes		
Incline dumbbell flyes	5	15
Incline dumbbell press	5	12
Flat bench dumbbell press	4	10
Leg raises	4	25

Note: The entire workout should be completed within 60 minutes

	Sets	Repetitions
Day 2: Back, cardio, abs		
Bicycle ride: 40 minutes		
Wide grip pull-ups	5	9
Close grip chin-ups	5	9
Dumbbell rows	5	10
Hanging leg raises	4	25

	Sets	Repetitions
Day 3: Shoulders, traps, cardio, calves		
Elliptical machine: 45 minutes		
Seated dumbbell shoulder press	5	10
Cable lateral raises	5	15
Bent-over dumbbell lateral raises	5	12
Barbell shrugs	4	10
Donkey calf raises	3	25

Day 4: Biceps, triceps, cardio, abs

	Sets	Repetitions
Standing barbell curl	5	12
Seated preacher curl	5	12
Lying triceps extension	5	12
Seated triceps dumbbell extension	5	12
Sit-ups	4	25

Outside run: 30 minutes

Day 5: Legs, calves, abs, cardio

	Sets	Repetitions
Jump rope: 30 minutes		
Leg extension	3	20
Leg curl	3	20
Squats	4	10
Stiff-leg dead lift	4	10
Lunges	3	10
Crunches	4	25

Day 6: Rest day
Day 7: Rest day

Four Days a Week
Duration: 60 minutes
Day 1: Back, biceps, abs, cardio

	Sets	Repetitions
Bent-over barbell rows	5	10
Wide grip pull-ups	5	10
Close grip pull-ups	5	10
Seated dumbbell concentration curls	5	12
Seated preacher curl	5	12

Inverted crunches	5	25
Full speed sprints	5	30 yards

Day 2: Chest, triceps, calves, cardio

Pec-dec machine	5	15
Dips	5	10
Dumbbell flat bench press	5	10
Close grip barbell bench press	5	12
Dumbbell triceps kick-backs	5	12
Crunches	5	25
Seated calf raises	3	20

Outside run: 30 minutes

Wednesday OFF

Day 3: Shoulders, traps, abs, cardio

	Sets	Repetitions
Cable lateral raises	5	15
Rear delt machine	5	15
Seated dumbbell shoulder press	5	10
Dumbbell shrugs	5	10
Leg raises	5	25

Swimming/running: 30 minutes

Day 4: Quadriceps, hamstrings, calves, cardio

	Sets	Repetitions
Leg extension	3	20
Leg curl	3	20
Squats	4	10
Stiff-leg dead lift	4	10
Lunges	2	10
Standing calf raises	3	20

Elliptical machine: 40 minutes

Day 5: Rest day
Day 6: Rest day
Day 7: Rest day

Three Days a Week
Day 1: Back, chest, abs, calves, cardio

	Sets	Repetitions
T-bar rows	5	10
Close grip chin-ups	5	10
Wide grip pull-ups	5	10
Cable cross-overs	5	15
Incline dumbbell press	5	10
Push-ups	5	25
Sit-ups	5	25
Seated calf raises	325	

Bicycle ride: 45 minutes

Day 2: Shoulders, biceps, triceps, abs, cardio

	Sets	Repetitions
Dumbbell shoulder press	5	10
Wide grip upright row	5	20
Bent-over dumbbell lateral raises	5	15
Dumbbell shrugs	5	10
Leg raises	5	25
Standing barbell curl	5	10
Standing hammer curls	5	12
Lying triceps extension	5	12
Cable triceps pushdown	5	15

Elliptical machine: 45 minutes

Day 3: Quadriceps, hamstrings, calves, abs, cardio

	Sets	Repetitions
Leg extension	3	20

Leg curl	3	20
Lunges	3	10
Hack squats	4	10
Stiff-leg dead lifts	3	10
Standing calf raises	3	25
Inverted crunches	5	25
Wind sprints	5	30 yards

Two Days a Week
Duration: 90 minutes
Day 1: Upper body

	Sets	Repetitions
Pull-ups	5	12
T-bar rows	5	12
Chin-ups	5	10
Incline dumbbell press	5	15
Incline dumbbell flyes	5	15
Dumbbell shoulder press	5	15
Lateral cable raises	5	15
Close grip upright rows	5	15
Sit-ups	3	25

Stationary bicycle: 30 minutes
Note: The entire workout should be completed within 90 minutes.

Day 2: Lower body

	Sets	Repetitions
Leg extension	4	20
Leg curl	4	20
Lunges	5	10
Squats	3	10
Stiff-leg dead lift	3	10
Standing calf raises	5	20
Hanging leg raises	5	20

Outside run: 30 minutes

One Day a Week

	Sets	Repetitions
Elliptical machine: 15 minutes		
Pec-dec machine	5	20
Incline dumbbell press	5	10
Pull-ups	5	10
T-bar rows	5	10
Standing barbell curl	5	10
Lying triceps extension	5	15
Dumbbell shoulder press	5	10
Upright row	5	10
Dumbbell lateral raises	5	15
Squats	5	12
Stiff-leg dead lift	5	12
Lunges	5	12
Standing calf raises	5	20
Crunches	3	25
Leg raises	3	25
Stationary bicycle: 15 minutes		

Note: The entire workout should be completed in 90 to 120 minutes.

Training Twice a Week

The twice per week full-body training regimen doesn't mean working out only two times a week. Instead, this is a way to exercise each major muscle group twice within a seven-day period. Each muscle will have approximately 72 hours of rest time in between workouts. Using the information I give you here, you can work each muscle group twice in a week by working out six, four, or only two times a week.

The advantages of this routine include "shocking the system," which means giving the body an immediate change in its exercise routine. These frequent changes help break stagnation and lead to increases in muscular strength and mass. This program also allows the body's weaker muscles extra attention by exercising them twice, instead of once, per week.

Mentally, you will feel invigorated by switching to a twice-per-week routine, because changing workouts from time to time adds enthusiasm to the training. This increases the fun factor, which leads to achieving a greater level of success.

Beginning Twice-Weekly Resistance Training Exercise
Six Days a Week

Day 1 and Day 4: Chest, shoulders, triceps, abs

	Sets	Repetitions
Standing cable cross-over	3	20
Barbell flat bench press	3	12
Shoulder press	3	12
Upright row	3	12
Triceps cable push-down	5	15
Sit-ups	3	10

Note: The entire workout should be completed in 60 minutes.

Day 2 and Day 5: Back, biceps, abs, cardio

Wide grip lat machine pull-down	3	10
Seated cable row	3	10
Dumbbell concentration curl	5	12
Crunches	3	10

Stationary bicycle: 20 minutes

Day 3 and Day 6: Legs, calves, abs, cardio

Leg extension	3	15
Leg curl	3	15
Lunges	3	10
Seated calf raise	3	15
Leg raises	3	10

Elliptical machine: 20 minutes

Four Days a Week
Duration: less than 60 minutes
Day 1 and Day 3: Upper body

	Sets	Repetitions
Incline barbell bench press	3	15
Decline barbell bench press	3	15
Wide grip lat machine pull-down	3	15
Seated cable row	3	15
Shoulder machine press	3	10
Upright row	3	10
Dumbbell curl	2	10
Triceps cable push-down	2	15
Crunches	2	10

Note: The entire workout should be completed in 60 minutes or less.

Day 2 and Day 4: Legs, abs, cardio

	Sets	Repetitions
Leg extension	3	15
Leg curl	3	15
Lunges	3	10
Sit-ups	2	10
Seated calf raise	2	15

Elliptical machine: 20 minutes

Two Days a Week
Day 1 and Day 2: Same routine for full body both days

	Sets	Repetitions
Incline bench press	3	12
Flat bench press	3	12
Wide grip lat machine pull-down	3	12
Seated cable row	3	12
Front shoulder press	3	10
Cable lateral raise	3	15

Preacher curl	3	12
Triceps pushdown	3	15

Stationary bicycle: 20 minutes

Leg extension	3	15
Leg curl	3	15
Lunges	3	10
Standing calf raises	2	15
Leg raises	2	10

Treadmill: 20 minutes

Note: The entire workout should be completed in 90 minutes or less.

Intermediate Twice-Weekly Resistance Training Program

Day 1 and Day 4: Chest, back, abs, cardio

	Sets	Repetitions
Incline dumbbell flyes	3	15
Incline barbell press	3	12
Decline barbell press	3	10
Close grip lat machine pull-down	3	12
Wide grip lat machine pull-down	3	10
Barbell row	3	10
Leg raises	3	15

Outside jog: 20 minutes

Note: The entire workout should be completed in 60 minutes or less.

Day 2 and Day 5: Shoulders, biceps, triceps, abs, cardio

	Sets	Repetitions
Cable lateral raises	3	15
Upright row	3	12
Shoulder press	3	10
Barbell curl	3	10
Preacher curl	3	12
Triceps cable push-down	3	15
Seated triceps extension	3	12
Inverted crunches	3	15

Day 3 and Day 6: Legs, calves, cardio

	Sets	Repetitions
Leg extension	3	20
Leg curl	3	20
Squats	3	10
Lunges	3	10
Standing calf raise	3	15

Elliptical machine: 30 minutes

Four Days a Week

Day 1 and Day 3: Upper body, cardio

	Sets	Repetitions
Barbell incline press	4	10
Barbell flat bench press	4	10
Wide-grip lat machine pull-down	4	10
Seated cable row	4	10
Front shoulder press	4	10
Upright row	4	10
Barbell curl	5	12
Lying triceps extension	5	12
Sit-ups	2	15

Elliptical machine: 30 minutes
Note: The entire workout should be completed in 75 minutes or less.

Day 2 and Day 4: Legs, calves, abs, cardio

	Sets	Repetitions
Leg extension	3	15
Leg curl	3	15
Leg press	3	10
Lunges	3	10
Seated calf raise	3	15

Stationary bicycle: 30 minutes

156 • GREAT BODY FOR SENIORS

Two Days a Week
Day 1: Upper body, cardio

	Sets	Repetitions
Pec-dec	5	15
Decline bench press	4	10
Wide grip lat machine pull-down	5	12
T-bar row	4	10
Shoulder press	5	10
Upright row	4	10
Cable curl	4	15
Dumbbell curl	3	10
Seated triceps extension	4	12
Inverted grip triceps cable push-down	3	15
Sit-ups	3	15

Stationary bicycle: 30 minutes

Note: The entire workout should be completed in 90 minutes or less.

Day 2: Lower body, abs, cardio

	Sets	Repetitions
Leg extension	4	15
Leg curl	4	15
Hack squat	4	10
Lunges	3	10
Standing calf raise	3	20

Elliptical machine: 30 minutes

Advanced Twice-Weekly Resistance Exercise Program

Six Days a Week
Day 1 and Day 4: Chest, back, abs, cardio

	Sets	Repetitions
Dumbbell incline flyes	3	15
Dumbbell incline press	3	12

	Sets	Repetitions
Dumbbell flat bench press	3	10
Pull-ups	5	10
Dumbbell row	3	10
T-bar row	4	10
Hanging leg raises	3	20

Outside jog: 30 minutes

Note: The entire workout should be completed in 75 minutes or less.

Day 2 and Day 5: Shoulders, biceps, triceps, abs, cardio

	Sets	Repetitions
Front shoulder press	4	10
Dumbbell lateral raise	4	12
Upright row	4	10
Barbell curl	4	10
Dumbbell curl	3	10
Lying triceps extension	4	12
Triceps kick-back	3	15
Side crunches	3	20

Treadmill: 30 minutes

Day 3 and Day 6: Legs, calves, abs, cardio

	Sets	Repetitions
Leg extension	4	20
Leg curl	4	20
Leg press	4	10
Lunges	4	12
Standing calf raise	3	15
Leg raises	3	20

Bicycle ride: 45 minutes

Four Days a Week

Day 1 and Day 3: Upper body, cardio

	Sets	Repetitions
Cable cross-over	4	15
Incline dumbbell press	4	10
Push-ups	3	15
Close grip lat machine pull-down	4	12
Wide grip lat machine pull-down	4	12
Dumbbell row	3	10
Front shoulder press	4	10
Dumbbell lateral raise	4	15
Upright row	3	10
Barbell curl	3	10
Preacher curl	3	10
Lying triceps extension	3	10
Seated triceps extension	3	12
Crunches	3	20

Outside run: 30 minutes

Note: The entire workout should be completed in 90 minutes or less.

Day 2 and Day 4: Lower body, abs, cardio

	Sets	Repetitions
Leg extension	4	20
Leg curl	4	20
Squats	4	10
Stiff-leg dead-lift	4	10
Lunges	3	10
Standing calf raises	3	20
Sit-ups	3	20
Wind sprints	5	30 yards

Two Days a Week
Day 1: Upper body, cardio

	Sets	Repetitions
Pec-dec	4	15
Incline dumbbell press	4	10
Dips	3	10
Pull-ups	4	10
Seated cable row	4	12
Dumbbell row	3	10
Barbell curl	4	12
Preacher curl	2	10
Shoulder press	5	10
Upright row	5	10
Lying triceps extension	4	15
Dumbbell triceps kick-back	3	12
Sit-ups	3	20

Treadmill: 45 minutes

Note: The entire workout should be completed in 120 minutes or less.

Day 2: Legs, calves, cardio, abs

	Sets	Repetitions
Leg extension	4	20
Leg curl	4	20
Front squats	4	10
Stiff-leg dead-lift	4	10
Standing calf raises	3	20
Crunches	3	20

Stationary bicycle: 45 minutes

Training Three Times Per Week

In the previous sections, I explained training regimens that included exercising each muscle group either once or twice per week within two to six days of exercise. In this chapter, I will discuss exercise routines that tone each major muscle group three times per week. For example, if you work out six days a week, you will exercise each muscle group three times within that period. If you exercise less often, you will still work each muscle group three times within your workout period.

This may seem to be too much strain on the muscles, with not enough rest time in between working the same muscle group. This isn't the case, because a minimum of 48 hours of rest is always allowed between exercising the same body part. Shocking the body by training it three times in one week will increase muscle endurance and recuperation time. Using this routine will give the best results when it's applied on a temporary basis, for several weeks or only a couple of months.

To avoid over-training, you will perform fewer sets per workout per muscle group. What I enjoy about this exercise routine is that, by training each muscle three times a week, you are constantly flushing blood through all of the major muscle areas. It's invigorating. However, after following this regimen for several weeks or months, you may begin to feel somewhat fatigued. You should then either reduce the number of sets per workout, or take one or two days off between workouts in order to rest.

Once you feel that this routine is losing its effectiveness and that you have reached a plateau or sticking point, then return back to training each muscle group either once or twice per week.

Beginner Three Times Weekly Weight Training
Six Days a Week
Day 1, Day 3, Day 5: Upper body, cardio

	Sets	Repetitions
Pec-dec	2	15
Barbell flat bench press	2	10
Wide grip lat machine pull-down	2	12
Seated cable row	2	10
Shoulder machine press	2	10

	Sets	Repetitions
Upright row	2	10
Cable curl	3	12
Triceps cable push-down	3	12
Ab machine	1	10

Stationary bicycle: 15 minutes

Note: The entire workout should be completed in 60 minutes or less

Day 2, Day 4, and Day 6: Legs, abs, cardio

	Sets	Repetitions
Leg press	2	10
Leg curl	2	15
Lunges	2	10
Seated calf raises	2	15
Seated ab machine	1	10

Elliptical machine: 15 minutes

Three Days a Week

Day 1, Day 2, and Day 3: Full body, cardio

	Sets	Repetitions
Flat bench press	3	10
Lat machine pull-down	3	12
Shoulder press	2	10
Upright row	2	10
Cable curl	2	10
Triceps cable push-down	2	10
Leg extension	2	12
Lug curl	2	12
Lunges	2	10
Standing calf raises	2	15
Sit-ups	2	10

Stair-stepper: 15 minutes

Note: The entire workout should be completed in 75 minutes or less.
[end table]

Intermediate Three Times Weekly Weight Training

Six days a week

Duration: less than 60 minutes

Day 1, day 2, and day 5: Upper body, cardio

	Sets	Repetitions
Incline cable flyes	4	15
Incline barbell press	3	12
Seated cable row	4	10
Lat machine pull-down	3	12
Dumbbell lateral raises	2	15
Shoulder press	3	10
Upright row	3	10
Preacher curl	5	10
Close grip bench press	5	10
Leg raises	2	10

Treadmill: 25 minutes

Note: The entire workout should be completed in 60 minutes or less.

Day 2, day 4, and day 6: Legs, abs, cardio

	Sets	Repetitions
Leg press	3	10
Leg extension	3	12
Leg curl	3	12
Lunges	3	10
Standing calf raises	2	15
Crunches	2	15

Bicycle ride: 25 minutes

Three Days a Week

Day 1, day 2, day 3: Full-body workout, cardio

	Sets	Repetitions
Flat bench press	4	10
Push-ups	3	12

Seated cable row	3	12
Lat machine pull-down	3	12
Dumbbell lateral raises	2	12
Shoulder press	2	10
Upright row	2	10
Dumbbell curl	3	10
Lying triceps extension	3	10
Hack squats	3	10
Leg curl	3	12
Lunges	3	10
Standing calf raise	2	15
Inverted crunches	2	15

Elliptical machine: 25 minutes

Note: The entire workout should be completed in 90 minutes or less.

Advanced Three Times Weekly Weight Training

Six Days a Week

Day 1, day 2, and day 5: Upper body, cardio

	Sets	Repetitions
Wide grip pull-ups	4	12
Seated cable row	4	12
Incline dumbbell press	4	12
Decline dumbbell press	4	12
Cable lateral raises	3	15
Upright row	3	10
Dumbbell shoulder press	2	10
Standing barbell curl	5	10
Seated triceps extension	5	12
Hanging leg raises	2	20

Outside run: 35 minutes

Note: The entire workout should be completed in 75 minutes or less.

Day 2, day 4, and day 6: Legs, abs, cardio

	Sets	Repetitions
Squats	3	10
Stiff-leg dead-lift	3	12
Hack squats	3	10
Lunges	3	10
Seated calf raises	2	20

Elliptical machine: 40 minutes

Three Days a Week

Day 1, day 2, and day 3: Full body workout, cardio

	Sets	Repetitions
Wide grip pull-ups	4	10
Dumbbell row	3	10
Incline dumbbell press	4	10
Incline flat bench press	3	10
Dumbbell shoulder press	3	10
Cable lateral raises	2	20
Upright row	2	15
Dumbbell curl	4	12
Seated triceps extension	4	12
Front squats	3	10
Stiff-leg dead-lift	3	10
Lunges	3	10
Standing calf raises	2	20

Treadmill: 40 minutes

Note: The entire workout should be completed in 90 minutes or less.

\

Chapter 13
Calisthenics Training

Calisthenics training is another form of resistance training. When most people think of resistance exercise routines, they immediately think of weight-lifting. Calisthenics exercises are actually another form of weight-lifting (resistance training). You use your own body weight as the resistance—in other words, you weight-lift yourself.

No matter which muscle you are exercising by lifting weights, there is always a way to exercise that same muscle but without weights. Instead, you use your own body weight as the resistance. The name for this is calisthenics, which comes from the ancient Greek words for beauty and strength.

Let's look at an example of how calisthenics is equivalent to weight training. Let's say you want to exercise your chest muscle. If you were weight-training, you would do bench presses. The calisthenics alternative would be push-ups. Instead of lat machine pull-downs to exercise the back muscles, you could perform pull-ups. Or rather than using the leg press machine, try either free squats or walking lunges to exercise the same muscles. Virtually every muscle in the body can be trained by either lifting weights or by lifting your own body weight.

If trained properly, a physique developed only through calisthenics can have a very impressive appearance. Usually, a body that was developed by weight training has a different appearance than one that was developed by calisthenics. The weight-trained physique may appear somewhat larger in mass, while the body weight-trained body would appear leaner and more well-defined. This is more of a natural and athletic look.

Calisthenics has other advantages, such as convenience. Regardless of where you are, you can always perform body-weight exercises. You don't need to be in the gym or need to use any form of equipment. In order to perform calisthenics, all you really need is yourself! Another advantage to calisthenics training is that people tend to sustain far fewer injuries. It's also good for people who for whatever reason aren't comfortable with the machines in a gym.

Basic Calisthenics Exercises

Chest: push-ups, dips
Back: pull-ups, chin-ups
Shoulders: Indian push-ups, inverted push-ups, body-weight shoulder press
Biceps: chin-ups
Triceps: diamond push-ups, dips
Legs: body-weight squats, lunges, single leg squats
Calves: standing calf raises
Abs: sit-ups, crunches, leg raises, hanging leg raises
Core: windshield wipers, planks
Neck: head raises, neck bridges

Beginning Calisthenics Training

Six Days a Week
Day 1, day 3, day 5: Upper body, cardio

	Sets	Repetitions
Wide grip pull-ups	3	10
Close grip chin-ups	3	10
Push-ups	3	10
Diamond push-ups	3	10
Sit-ups	3	10

Stationary bicycle: 20 minutes
Note: The entire workout should be completed in 45 minutes or less.

Day 2, day 4, and day 6: Legs, abs, cardio

	Sets	Repetitions
Body squats	5	15
Lunges	5	15
Standing calf raises	3	25
Crunches	3	15

Treadmill: 20 minutes

Note: The entire workout should be completed in 45 minutes or less.

Five Days a Week
Day 1: Upper body

	Sets	Repetitions
Push-ups	3	10
Pull-ups	3	10
Sit-ups	3	10

Note: The entire workout should take 20 minutes or less.

Day 2: Legs, abs

	Sets	Repetitions
Lunges	3	10
Body squats	3	15
Standing calf raises	3	20
Crunches	3	10

Note: The entire workout should take 20 minutes or less.

Day 3: Upper body

	Sets	Repetitions
Push-ups	3	10
Chin-ups	3	10
Leg raises	3	10

Note: The entire workout should take 20 minutes or less.

Day 4: Legs, abs

	Sets	Repetitions
Body squats	3	15
Lunges	3	10
Crunches	3	10

Note: The entire workout should take 20 minutes or less.

Day 5: Full body

	Sets	Repetitions
Wide grip pull-ups	3	10
Dips	3	10
Lunges	3	10
Body squats	3	10
Sit-ups	3	10
Standing calf raises	3	10

Note: The entire workout should take 20 minutes or less.

Four Days a Week

Day 1 and day 3: Upper body

	Sets	Repetitions
Dips	3	10
Push-ups	2	10
Wide grip pull-ups	3	10
Close grip chin-ups	2	10
Crunches	3	10

Note: The entire workout should be completed in 25 minutes or less.

Day 2 and day 4: Legs, abs

	Sets	Repetitions
Lunges	4	10
Body squats	4	15
Standing calf raises	3	20
Sit-ups	4	10

Note: The entire workout should be completed in 25 minutes or less.

Three Days a Week
Day 1, day 2, and day 3: Full body

	Sets	Repetitions
Wide grip pull-ups	3	10
Chin-ups	3	10
Push-ups	3	10
Dips	3	10
Lunges	3	10
Body squats	3	10
Standing calf raises	3	20
Sit-ups	3	10

Note: The entire workout should be completed in 40 minutes or less.

Two Days a Week
Day 1: Upper body

	Sets	Repetitions
Close grip pull-ups	4	10
Chin-ups	3	10
Diamond push-ups	4	10
Push-ups	3	10
Sit-ups	2	10

Note: The entire workout should be completed in 30 minutes or less.

Day 2: Legs, abs

	Sets	Repetitions
Lunges	4	10
Free squats	4	10
Standing calf raises	4	25
Crunches	3	10

Note: The entire workout should be completed in 30 minutes or less.

One Day a Week
Day 1: Full body

	Sets	Repetitions
Wide grip pull-ups	4	10
Chin-ups	4	10
Diamond push-ups	4	10
Push-ups	4	10
Free squats	4	15
Lunges	4	10
Standing calf raises	4	20
Crunches	4	10

Note: The entire workout should be completed in 45 minutes or less.

Intermediate Calisthenics Training

Five Days a Week
Day 1, day 3, day 5: Upper body, cardio

	Sets	Repetitions
Push-ups	4	15
Dips	3	15
Pull-ups	4	12
Chin-ups	3	12
Indian push-ups	4	10
Leg raises	2	15

Elliptical machine: 25 minutes
Note: The entire workout should be completed in 60 minutes or less.

Day 2, day 4, day 6: Legs, abs, cardio

	Sets	Repetitions
Free squats	4	20
Lunges	4	15
Standing calf raises	3	10
Crunches	2	15

Stationary bicycle: 25 minutes

Note: The entire workout should be completed in 60 minutes or less.

Five Days a Week
Day 1, day 3: Upper body, cardio

	Sets	Repetitions
Push-ups	4	15
Diamond push-ups	3	10
Indian push-ups	3	10
Pull-ups	4	12
Chin-ups	3	12
Leg raises	3	15

Treadmill: 25 minutes

Note: The entire workout should be completed in 60 minutes or less.

Day 2, day 4: Legs, cardio

	Sets	Repetitions
Free squats	5	15
Lunges	5	15
Standing calf raises	4	20
Crunches	3	15

Stationary bicycle: 25 minutes

Note: The entire workout should be completed in 60 minutes or less.

Day 5: Full body

	Sets	Repetitions
Push-ups	5	15
Pull-ups	5	12
Indian push-ups	3	10
Free squats	4	15
Lunges	4	15
Standing calf raises	3	20
Sit-ups	3	15

Elliptical machine: 25 minutes

Note: The entire workout should be completed in 60 minutes or less.

Four Days a Week
Day 1, day 4: Upper body, cardio

	Sets	Repetitions
Push-ups	4	15
Dips	4	12
Indian push-ups	3	10
Wide grip pull-ups	4	12
Chin-ups	4	12
Inverted crunches	3	15

Elliptical machine: 25 minutes
Note: The entire workout should be completed in 75 minutes or less.

Day 2, day 4: Legs, abs, cardio

	Sets	Repetitions
Free squats	5	15
Lunges	5	12
Standing calf raises	3	20

Stationary bicycle: 25 minutes
Note: The entire workout should be completed in 75 minutes or less.

Three Days a Week
Day 1, day 2, day 3: Full body, cardio

	Sets	Repetitions
Push-ups	4	15
Dips	2	12
Pull-ups	4	12
Chin-ups	2	12
Indian push-ups	3	10
Free squats	4	15
Lunges	2	10
Standing calf raises	3	15
Crunches	3	15

Stationary bicycle: 25 minutes
Note: The entire workout should be completed in 75 minutes or less.

Two Days a Week
Day 1: Upper body, cardio

	Sets	Repetitions
Push-ups	5	12
Dips	5	12
Wide grip pull-ups	5	12
Chin-ups	5	12
Indian push-ups	4	10
Sit-ups	4	15

Elliptical machine: 25 minutes
Note: The entire workout should be completed in 75 minutes or less.

Day 2: Legs, abs, cardio

	Sets	Repetitions
Lunges	6	12
Free squats	6	12
Standing calf raises	5	20
Crunches	4	15

Stationary bicycle: 25 minutes
Note: The entire workout should be completed in 75 minutes or less.

One Day a Week
Day 1: Full body, cardio

	Sets	Repetitions
Push-ups	5	12
Dips	5	12
Wide grip pull-ups	5	12
Chin-ups	5	12
Indian push-ups	4	10
Free squats	6	12
Lunges	6	12
Standing calf raises	5	20
Sit-ups	5	15

Treadmill: 25 minutes

Note: The entire workout should be completed in 90 minutes or less.

Advanced Calisthenics Training

Six Days a Week

Day 1, day 2, day 5: Upper body, cardio

	Sets	Repetitions
Wide grip pull-ups	5	12
Chin-ups	4	12
Dips	5	12
Push-ups	4	15
Shoulder press	4	10
Indian push-ups	3	12
Hanging leg raises	5	15

Treadmill: 40 minutes

Note: The entire workout should be completed in 75 minutes or less.

Day 2, day 4, and day 6: Legs, abs, cardio

	Sets	Repetitions
Free squats	5	15
Lunges	5	15
Standing calf raises	4	20
Crunches	5	20

Bicycle ride: 40 minutes

Note: The entire workout should be completed in 75 minutes or less.

Five Days a Week

Day 2, day 3: Upper body, cardio

	Sets	Repetitions
Pull-ups	5	12
Chin-ups	4	12
Dips	5	12
Push-ups	4	15

	Sets	Repetitions
Shoulder press	4	10
Indian push-ups	4	10
Crunches	3	20

Elliptical machine: 40 minutes

Note: The entire workout should be completed in 75 minutes or less.

Day 2 and day 4: Legs, abs, cardio

	Sets	Repetitions
Lunges	5	12
Free squats	5	15
Standing calf raises	4	20
Sit-ups	3	20

Treadmill: 40 minutes

Note: The entire workout should be completed in 75 minutes or less.

Day 5: Full body, cardio

	Sets	Repetitions
Pull-ups	3	12
Chin-ups	4	10
Dips	3	10
Push-ups	4	15
Inverted shoulder press	2	8
Indian push-ups	2	10
Free squats	4	12
Lunges	3	10
Standing calf raises	3	20
Hanging leg raises	3	12

Outside jog: 30 minutes

Note: The entire workout should be completed in 75 minutes or less.

Four Days a Week
Day 1, day 3: Upper body, cardio

	Sets	Repetitions
Pull-ups	4	12
Chin-ups	5	10
Dips	4	12
Push-ups	5	12
Inverted shoulder presses	4	8
Indian push-ups	5	10
Hanging leg raises	3	15

Treadmill: 40 minutes
Note: The entire workout should be completed in 75 minutes or less.

Day 2, day 4: Legs, abs, cardio

	Sets	Repetitions
Free squats	5	15
Lunges	5	15
Standing calf raises	4	20
Sit-ups	3	15

Bicycle ride: 40 minutes
Note: The entire workout should be completed in 75 minutes or less.

Three Days a Week
Day 1, day 2, day 3: Full body, cardio

	Sets	Repetitions
Push-ups	4	12
Diamond push-ups	3	10
Pull-ups	4	10
Chin-ups	3	10
Indian push-ups	3	10
Inverted shoulder press	2	8
Lunges	4	12
Free squats	4	15

	Sets	Repetitions
Standing calf raises	3	20
Leg raises	3	15

Treadmill: 40 minutes

Note: The entire workout should be completed in 90 minutes or less.

Two Days a Week
Day 1: Upper body, cardio

	Sets	Repetitions
Push-ups	6	15
Dips	6	15
Pull-ups	6	12
Chin-ups	6	12
Body weight shoulder press	5	8
Indian push-ups	5	10
Crunches	4	20

Bicycle ride: 40 minutes

Note: The entire workout should be completed in 75 minutes or less.

Day 2: Legs, abs, cardio

	Sets	Repetitions
Lunges	7	10
Free squats	7	15
Standing calf raises	5	25
Sit-ups	4	20

Elliptical machine: 40 minutes

Note: The entire workout should be completed in 75 minutes or less.

One Day a Week
Day 1: Full body, cardio

	Sets	Repetitions
Dips	4	12
Diamond push-ups	3	10
Push-ups	4	15

Wide grip pull-ups	4	10
Close grip pull-ups	3	12
Chin-ups	4	10
Indian push-ups	4	10
Body weight shoulder press	4	8
Free squats	6	20
Lunges	6	12
Standing calf raises	5	20

Stationary bicycle: 40 minutes

Note: The entire workout should be completed in 90 minutes or less.

Chapter 14
Supersetting

There are many different exercise routines, and each and every one of them has their advantages. Choosing a workout regimen that is conducive to your lifestyle is very important. For this reason, I have written many different workouts in order for you to choose which one best fits your schedule.

Supersetting workouts are different because there is virtually no rest time in between exercises. The cardiovascular effect this creates is simultaneously added to the resistance exercise, giving you a more intense workout.

Another advantage to supersetting exercises is that the workouts are completed in a shorter amount of time. This type of training is conducive to those that have limited time to exercise. Within a shorter amount of time, you complete a full resistance and cardiovascular routine simultaneously. Cardiovascular training includes raising the body's heart rate. When the heart rate is elevated, you can begin to feel a shortness of breath. Most people experience this via running, bicycling, and playing sports. However, you can also increase your heart rate when performing resistance training by supersetting, because there is no rest time in between sets. Superset training is a very efficient way to train.

Beginner Superset Training
Six Days a Week
Day 1, day 4: Chest, back, abs

	Sets	Repetitions
Barbell bench press supersetted with lat machine pull-down	5	10
Sit-ups supersetted with crunches	2	10

Note: The entire routine should be completed in 20 minutes or less.

Day 2, day 6: Shoulders, triceps, biceps

	Sets	Repetitions
Shoulder press supersetted with dumbbell lateral raises	3	10
Triceps cable push-downs supersetted with barbell curls	3	10

Note: The entire routine should be completed in 20 minutes or less.

Day 3, day 6: Legs, abs

	Sets	Repetitions
Leg extensions supersetted with leg curls	4	12
Crunches supersetted with seated calf raises	3	10

Note: The entire routine should be completed in 20 minutes or less.

Five Days a Week

Day 1, day 3: Chest, back, shoulders, abs

	Sets	Repetitions
Incline barbell press supersetted with lat machine pull-downs	5	10
Upright rows supersetted with shoulder presses	3	10
Sit-ups supersetted with crunches	2	15

Note: The entire workout should be completed in 20 minutes or less.

Day 2, day 4: Legs, abs, triceps, biceps

	Sets	Repetitions
Leg extensions supersetted with leg curls	5	15

Barbell curls supersetted with
    triceps cable push-downs   3   12
Standing calf raises supersetted with crunches   3   15

Note: The entire workout should be completed in 20 minutes or less.

Four Days a Week
Day 1, day 3: Chest, shoulders, back, abs

	Sets	*Repetitions*
Barbell bench press supersetted with lat machine pull-downs	5	10
Upright rows supersetted with shoulder presses	3	10
Sit-ups supersetted with crunches	2	10

Day 2, day 4: Legs, abs, biceps, triceps
Note: The entire workout should be completed in 15 minutes or less.

	Sets	*Repetitions*
Leg extensions supersetted with leg curls	5	15
Seated calf raises supersetted with crunches	3	15
Standing barbell curl supersetted with triceps cable push-downs	3	12

Note: The entire workout should be completed in 15 minutes or less.

Three Days a Week
Day 1, day 2, day 3: full body

	Sets	*Repetitions*
Incline barbell press supersetted with wide grip lat machine pull-downs	5	12
Dumbbell curls supersetted with seated triceps extension	3	12
Upright row supersetted with shoulder press	3	10
Leg extensions supersetted with leg curls	5	12
Sit-ups supersetted with seated calf raises	3	12

Note: The entire workout should be completed in 20 minutes or less.

Two Days a Week
Day 1, day 2: Full body

	Sets	Repetitions
Barbell bench press supersetted with lat machine pull-downs	5	12
Upright rows supersetted with shoulder presses	3	10
Dumbbell concentration curls supersetted with triceps cable push-downs	3	12
Leg extensions supersetted with leg curls	5	12
Standing calf raises supersetted with sit-ups	3	15

Note: The entire workout should be completed in 20 minutes or less.

One Day a Week
Day 1: full body

	Sets	Repetitions
Barbell bench press supersetted with lat machine pull-downs	5	10
Upright rows supersetted with shoulder presses	3	10
Dumbbell curls supersetted with triceps cable push-downs	3	10
Leg extensions supersetted with leg curls	5	12
Seated calf raises supersetted with crunches	3	15

Note: The entire workout should be completed in 20 minutes or less.

Intermediate Superset Resistance Training

Six Days a Week
Day 1, day 4: Chest, back, abs, cardio

	Sets	Repetitions
Pec-dec supersetted with dumbbell press	4	12

	Sets	Repetitions
Lat machine pull-downs supersetted with seated cable rows	4	12
Crunches supersetted with leg raises	3	15

Elliptical machine: 20 minutes

Note: The entire workout should be complete in 40 minutes or less.

Day 2, day 5: Shoulders, biceps, triceps, abs, cardio

	Sets	Repetitions
Upright rows supersetted with shoulder presses	6	10
Barbell curls supersetted with lying triceps extensions	4	12
Leg raises supersetted with inverted crunches	3	15

Treadmill: 20 minutes

Note: The entire workout should be complete in 40 minutes or less.

Day 3, day 6: Legs, abs, cardio

	Sets	Repetitions
Leg press supersetted with leg curls	4	12
Lunges supersetted with sit-ups	3	12

Stationary bicycle: 20 minutes

Note: The entire workout should be complete in 40 minutes or less.

Five Days a Week

Day 1, day 3: Chest, back, shoulders, abs, cardio

	Sets	Repetitions
Cable crossovers supersetted with dumbbell incline press	3	12
Lat machine pull-down supersetted with T-bar rows	3	12
Upright rows supersetted with dumbbell shoulder press	5	10
Crunches supersetted with leg raises	3	15

Bicycle ride: 25 minutes
Note: The entire workout should be completed in 40 minutes or less.

Day 2, day 4: Legs, biceps, triceps, abs, cardio

	Sets	Repetitions
Leg extensions supersetted with hack squats	3	12
Leg curls supersetted with sit-ups	3	12
Dumbbell curls supersetted with close grip bench press	5	12
Seated calf raises supersetted with standing calf raises	2	15
Sprints	5	30 yards

Note: The entire workout should be completed in 40 minutes or less.

Day 5: Full body, cardio

	Sets	Repetitions
Lat machine pull-down s upersetted with pec-dec	3	15
Seated cable rows supersetted with incline barbell press	3	15
Upright rows supersetted with shoulder presses	3	15
Barbell curls supersetted with seated triceps extensions	3	15
Leg press supersetted with leg curls	3	15
Leg extensions supersetted with crunches	3	16
Seated calf raises supersetted with standing calf raises	2	15

Stationary bicycle: 25 minutes
Note: The entire workout should be completed in 40 minutes or less.

Four Days a Week
Day 1, day 3: Chest, back, shoulders, abs, cardio

	Sets	Repetitions
Dumbbell flyes supersetted with incline press	5	12
Lat machine pull-downs supersetted with T-bar rows	5	12
Lateral raises supersetted with shoulder presses	5	12
Leg raises supersetted with crunches	2	15

Outside jog: 25 minutes
Note: The entire workout should be completed in 50 minutes or less.

Day 2, day 4: Legs, biceps, triceps, cardio

	Sets	Repetitions
Hack squats supersetted with leg curls	5	12
Barbell curls supersetted with lying triceps extensions	4	12
Standing calf raises supersetted with sit-ups	3	15

Elliptical machine: 25 minutes
Note: The entire workout should be completed in 50 minutes or less.

Three Days a Week
Day 1, day 2, day 3: full body, cardio

	Sets	Repetitions
Lat machine pull-downs supersetted with incline bench press	3	15
seated cable rows supersetted with pec-dec	3	15
upright rows supersetted with dumbbell lateral raises	3	15
Shoulder press supersetted with bent-over cable lateral raises	3	15
Dumbbell curls supersetted with seated triceps extensions	5	15

Leg presses supersetted with leg curls	3	15
Lunges supersetted with standing calf raises	3	15
Sit-ups supersetted with leg raises	3	15
Outside jog: 30 minutes		

Note: The entire workout should be completed in 60 minutes or less.

Two Days a Week
Day 1, day 2: full body and cardio

	Sets	Repetitions
Incline barbell press supersetted with T-bar rows	3	20
Cable crossovers supersetted with lat machine pull-downs	3	20
Dumbbell lateral raises supersetted with shoulder presses	3	20
Upright rows supersetted with bent-over lateral raises	3	20
Preacher curls supersetted with triceps kick-backs	3	20
Hack squats supersetted with leg curls	3	20
Lunges supersetted with standing calf raises	3	20
Crunches supersetted with sit-ups	3	20
Sprints	5	25 yards

Note: The entire workout should be completed in 60 minutes or less.

One Day a Week
Day 1: full body, cardio

	Sets	Repetitions
Pec-dec supersetted with seated cable rows	3	10
Incline barbell press supersetted with lat machine pull-down	3	10

Dumbbell lateral raises supersetted with upright rows	3	10
Shoulder presses supersetted with bent-over lateral raises	3	10
Dumbbell concentration curls supersetted with lying triceps extensions	3	10
Leg extensions supersetted with leg curls	3	10
Lunges supersetted with leg presses	3	10
Standing calf raises supersetted with crunches	3	20

Stationary bicycle: 30 minutes

Note: The entire workout should be completed in 60 minutes or less.

Advanced Superset Resistance Training

Six Days a Week

Day 1, day 3, day 5: Upper body, cardio

	Sets	Repetitions
Cable cross-overs supersetted with pull-ups	3	10
Incline barbell press supersetted with lat machine pull-downs	3	12
Dips supersetted with seated cable rows	3	12
Shoulder presses supersetted with dumbbell lateral raises	2	12
Upright rows supersetted with bent-over lateral raises	3	12
Barbell curls supersetted with lying triceps extensions	3	15
Hanging leg raises supersetted with inverted crunches	2	15

Outside jog: 30 minutes

Note: The entire workout should be completed in 75 minutes or less.

188 • GREAT BODY FOR SENIORS

Day 2, day 4, day 6: Legs, abs, cardio

	Sets	Repetitions
Leg extensions supersetted with leg curls	3	15
Squats supersetted with stiff-leg dead-lifts	3	12
Standing calf raises supersetted with seated calf raises	2	15
Sit-ups supersetted with crunches	2	15

Bicycle ride: 30 minutes

Note: The entire workout should be completed in 75 minutes or less.

Five Days a Week

Day 1, day 3: Upper body, cardio

	Sets	Repetitions
Push-ups supersetted with incline barbell press	3	15
Pec-deck supersetted with lat machine pull-downs	3	15
Dumbbell rows supersetted with pull-ups	3	12
Shoulder presses supersetted with upright rows	3	12
Bent-over lateral raises supersetted with front raises	2	12
Dumbbell concentration curls supersetted with seated triceps extensions	3	15
Hanging leg raises supersetted with crunches	2	15

Treadmill: 30 minutes

Note: The entire workout should be completed in 75 minutes or less.

Day 2, day 4: Legs, abs, cardio

	Sets	Repetitions
Leg extensions supersetted with leg curls	3	15
Hack squats supersetted with lunges	3	10

	Sets	Repetitions
Seated calf raises supersetted with standing calf raises	2	15
Inverted crunches supersetted with crunches	2	15
Sprints	6	30 yards

Note: The entire workout should be completed in 75 minutes or less.

Day 5: Full body, cardio

	Sets	Repetitions
Incline barbell press supersetted with pull-ups	2	12
Dumbbell flyes supersetted with lat machine pull-downs	2	12
Dips supersetted with dumbbell rows	2	12
Shoulder press supersetted with upright rows	2	12
Dumbbell lateral raises supersetted with bent-over lateral raises	2	12
Preacher curls supersetted with dumbbell triceps kick-backs	2	12
Lunges supersetted with leg curls	2	12
Squats supersetted with stiff-leg dead-lifts	2	12
Sit-ups supersetted with leg raises	2	15
Bicycle ride: 30 minutes		

Note: The entire workout should be completed in 75 minutes or less.

Four Days a Week

Day 1, day 3: Upper body, cardio

	Sets	Repetitions
Cable cross-overs supersetted with pull-ups	3	12
Incline dumbbell press supersetted with lat machine pull-downs	3	15
Push-ups supersetted with dumbbell rows	3	12
Upright rows supersetted with dumbbell shoulder presses	3	10

Lateral raises supersetted with
    bent-over lateral raises 2 12
Preacher curls supersetted
    with seated triceps extensions 3 12
Inverted crunches supersetted with crunches 2 15
Sprints 5 30 yards

Note: The entire workout should be completed in 75 minutes or less.

Day 2, day 4: Legs, abs, cardio

	Sets	Repetitions
Leg extensions supersetted with leg curls	3	12
Lunges supersetted with squats	3	12
Standing calf raises supersetted with seated calf raises	2	15
Leg raises supersetted with sit-ups	2	15

Treadmill: 30 minutes

Note: The entire workout should be completed in 75 minutes or less.

Three Days a Week

Day 1, day 2, day 3: full body, cardio

	Sets	Repetitions
Push-ups supersetted with lat machine pull-downs	3	10
Incline dumbbell press supersetted with pull-ups	2	10
Dips supersetted with dumbbell rows	2	10
Upright rows supersetted with dumbbell shoulder presses	3	10
Lateral raises supersetted with bent-over lateral raises	2	10
Preacher curls supersetted with triceps kick-backs	4	10
Lunges supersetted with leg curls	3	10

	Sets	Repetitions
Squats supersetted with stiff-leg dead-lifts	2	10
Standing calf raises supersetted with leg raises	3	15

Outside jog: 30 minutes

Note: The entire workout should be completed in 75 minutes or less.

Two Days a Week
Day 1, day 2: full body, cardio

	Sets	Repetitions
Incline dumbbell press supersetted with seated cable rows	3	15
Cable cross-overs supersetted with pull-ups	3	10
Push-ups supersetted with dumbbell rows	2	12
Dumbbell shoulder presses supersetted with dumbbell lateral raises	3	15
Upright rows supersetted with bent-over lateral raises	3	15
Preacher curls supersetted with seated triceps extensions	4	15
Leg curls supersetted with hack squats	3	12
Lunges supersetted with leg presses	3	15
Seated calf raises supersetted with hanging leg raises	4	15

Outside bicycle ride: 30 minutes

Note: The entire workout should be completed in 75 minutes or less.

One Day a Week
Day 1: full body, cardio

	Sets	Repetitions
Cable crossovers supersetted with pull-ups	3	8
Incline barbell presses supersetted with seated cable rows	3	8

Dips supersetted with dumbbell rows	3	8
Upright rows supersetted with dumbbell shoulder presses	3	8
Lateral raises supersetted with bent-over lateral raises	3	8
Barbell curls supersetted with close-grip bench press	5	8
Leg extensions supersetted with leg curls	3	8
Squats supersetted with stiff-leg dead-lifts	3	8
Lunges supersetted with sit-ups	3	8
Seated calf raises supersetted with crunches	3	8

Outside jog: 30 minutes

Note: The entire workout should be completed in 75 minutes or less.

Beginning Calisthenics Superset Training

Six Days a Week

Day 1, day 2, day 5: Upper body

	Sets	Repetitions
Push-ups supersetted with pull-ups	2	12
Diamond push-ups supersetted with chin-ups	2	12
Sit-ups supersetted with crunches	2	10

Note: The entire workout should be completed in 15 minutes or less.

Day 2, day 4, day 6: Legs, abs

	Sets	Repetitions
Lunges supersetted with free squats	3	15
Sit-ups supersetted with standing calf raises	3	15

Note: The entire workout should be completed in 15 minutes or less.

Five Days a Week

Day 1, day 3: Upper body

	Sets	Repetitions
Push-ups supersetted with pull-ups	2	12
Diamond push-ups supersetted with chin-ups	2	12
Crunches supersetted with leg-raises	2	10

Note: The entire workout should be completed in 15 minutes or less.

Day 2, day 4: Legs, abs

	Sets	Repetitions
Lunges supersetted with free squats	3	15
Crunches supersetted with standing calf raises	2	15

Note: The entire workout should be completed in 15 minutes or less.

Day 5: Full body

	Sets	Repetitions
Diamond push-ups supersetted with chin-ups	2	8
Push-ups supersetted with pull-ups	1	8
Free squats supersetted with lunges	3	15
Standing calf raises supersetted with sit-ups	3	15

Note: The entire workout should be completed in 15 minutes or less.

Four Days a Week

Day 1, day 3: Upper body

	Sets	Repetitions
Pull-ups supersetted with push-ups	3	8
Chin-ups supersetted with diamond push-ups	3	8
Crunches supersetted with sit-ups	2	12

Note: The entire workout should be completed in 15 minutes or less.

Day 2, day 4: Legs, abs

	Sets	Repetitions
Lunges supersetted with free squats	3	15
Standing calf raises supersetted with crunches	3	15

Note: The entire workout should be completed in 15 minutes or less.

Three Days a Week
Day 1, day 2, day 3: full body

	Sets	Repetitions
Pull-ups supersetted with push-ups	3	8
Chin-ups supersetted with diamond push-ups	3	8
Lunges supersetted with free squats	3	12
Standing calf raises supersetted with crunches	3	15

Note: The entire workout should be completed in 20 minutes or less.

Two Days a Week
Day 1, day 2: full body

	Sets	Repetitions
Chin-ups supersetted with diamond push-ups	3	10
Pull-ups supersetted with push-ups	3	10
Lunges supersetted with free squats	3	15
Standing calf raises supersetted with crunches	3	15

Note: The entire workout should be completed in 20 minutes or less.

One Day a Week
Day 1: full body

	Sets	Repetitions
Push-ups supersetted with pull-ups	3	10
Diamond push-ups supersetted with chin-ups	3	10
Free squats supersetted with lunges	3	15
Standing calf raises supersetted with sit-ups	3	15

Note: The entire workout should be completed in 20 minutes or less.

Intermediate Calisthenics Superset Training

Six Days a Week

Day 1, day 3, day 5: Upper body, cardio

	Sets	Repetitions
Pull-ups supersetted with push-ups	3	12
Chin-ups supersetted with diamond push-ups	3	12
Indian push-ups supersetted with dips	3	10
Leg raises supersetted with crunches	2	15

Elliptical machine: 20 minutes

Note: The entire workout should be completed in 40 minutes or less.

Day 2, day 4, day 6: Legs, abs, cardio

	Sets	Repetitions
Free squats supersetted with lunges	3	20
Plyometric jump squats supersetted with standing calf raises	3	20
Sit-ups supersetted with inverted crunches	2	15

Treadmill: 20 minutes

Note: The entire workout should be completed in 40 minutes or less.

Five Days a Week

Day 1, day 3: upper body, cardio

	Sets	Repetitions
Pull-ups supersetted with push-ups	3	10
Chin-ups supersetted with diamond push-ups	3	10
Indian push-ups supersetted with dips	3	10
Sit-ups supersetted with crunches	2	15

Treadmill: 20 minutes

Note: The entire workout should be completed in 40 minutes or less.

Day 2, day 4: Legs, abs, cardio

	Sets	Repetitions
Lunges supersetted with free squats	3	15
Plyometric jump squats supersetted with standing calf raises	3	15
Leg raises supersetted with inverted crunches	2	15

Stationary bicycle: 20 minutes

Note: The entire workout should be completed in 40 minutes or less.

Day 5: Full body, cardio

	Sets	Repetitions
Pull-ups supersetted with push-ups	3	12
Chin-ups supersetted with diamond push-ups	3	12
Indian push-ups supersetted with dips	3	12
Free squats supersetted with plyometric jump squats	3	15
Lunges supersetted with crunches	3	12
Standing calf raises supersetted with sit-ups	2	15

Elliptical machine: 20 minutes

Note: The entire workout should be completed in 40 minutes or less.

Four Days a Week

Day 1, day 3, day 4: full body, cardio

	Sets	Repetitions
Chin-ups supersetted with diamond push-ups	3	9
Pull-ups supersetted with dips	2	9
Indian push-ups supersetted with push-ups	3	9
Lunges supersetted with plyometric jump squats	2	12
Free squats supersetted with crunches	3	15
Standing calf raises supersetted with leg-raises	2	12

Elliptical machine: 20 minutes

Note: The entire workout should be completed in 40 minutes or less.

Three Days a Week

Day 1, day 2, day 3: Full body, cardio

	Sets	Repetitions
Push-ups supersetted with Indian push-ups	3	10
Dips supersetted with chin-ups	3	10
Diamond push-ups supersetted with pull-ups	3	10
Free squats supersetted with plyometric jump squats	3	12
Lunges supersetted with standing calf raises	3	12
Sit-ups supersetted with crunches	2	16

Stationary bicycle: 20 minutes

Note: The entire workout should be completed in 40 minutes or less.

Two Days a Week

Day 1, day 2: Full body, cardio

	Sets	Repetitions
Push-ups supersetted with pull-ups	4	12
Diamond push-ups supersetted with chin-ups	4	12
Indian push-ups supersetted with dips	3	12
Free squats supersetted with plyometric jump squats	3	12
Lunges supersetted with standing calf raises	3	15
Crunches supersetted with leg raises	2	15

Stationary bicycle: 20 minutes

Note: The entire workout should be completed in 50 minutes or less.

One Day a Week

	Sets	Repetitions
Pull-ups supersetted with dips	4	10
Chin-ups supersetted with diamond push-ups	4	10

Indian push-ups supersetted with push-ups	4	10
Free squats supersetted with lunges	4	10
Plyometric jump squats supersetted with crunches	3	10
Standing calf raises supersetted with leg-raises	3	10

Elliptical machine: 20 minutes

Note: The entire workout should be completed in 60 minutes or less.

Advanced Calisthenics Superset Training

Six Days a Week

Day 1, day 2, day 4: Upper body, cardio

	Sets	*Repetitions*
Push-ups supersetted with pull-ups	4	12
Dips supersetted with chin-ups	4	12
Indian push-ups supersetted with body weight shoulder presses	3	10
Hanging leg-raises supersetted with crunches	3	20

Outside jog: 30 minutes

Note: The entire workout should be completed in 60 minutes or less.

Day 2, day 4, day 6: Legs, cardio

	Sets	*Repetitions*
Free squats supersetted with plyometric jump squats	4	15
Lunges supersetted with single leg squats	4	12
Crunches supersetted with standing calf raises	4	20
Sprints	5	30 yards

Note: The entire workout should be completed in 60 minutes or less.

Five Days a Week

Day 1, day 3: Upper body, cardio

	Sets	*Repetitions*
Push-ups supersetted with pull-ups	4	10

Dips supersetted with chin-ups	4	10
Indian push-ups supersetted with body weight shoulder presses	3	8
Hanging leg raises supersetted with crunches	3	20

Treadmill: 30 minutes
Note: The entire workout should be completed in 60 minutes or less.

Day 2, day 4: Legs, cardio

	Sets	Repetitions
Plyometric jump squats supersetted with free squats	4	15
Single leg squats supersetted with lunges	4	15
Standing calf raises supersetted with crunches	4	20

Bicycle ride: 30 minutes
Note: The entire workout should be completed in 60 minutes or less.

Day 5: full body, cardio

	Sets	Repetitions
Dips supersetted with chin-ups	3	12
Push-ups supersetted with pull-ups	3	12
Indian push-ups supersetted with body weight shoulder presses	3	12
Sit-ups supersetted with standing calf raises	3	15
Plyometric jump squats supersetted with free squats	3	15
Single leg squats supersetted with lunges	3	12

Outside jog: 20 minutes
Note: The entire workout should be completed in 60 minutes or less.

Four Days a Week
Day 1, day 2, day 3, day 4: full body, cardio

	Sets	Repetitions
Chin-ups supersetted with dips	3	10

	Sets	Repetitions
Pull-ups supersetted with push-ups	3	10
Body weight shoulder presses supersetted with Indian push-ups	3	10
Free squats supersetted with plyometric jump squats	3	10
Lunges supersetted with single leg squats	3	10
Hanging leg raises supersetted with standing calf raises	3	10

Treadmill: 30 minutes

Note: The entire workout should be completed in 60 minutes or less.

Three Days a Week
Day, day 2, day3: full body, cardio

	Sets	Repetitions
Dips supersetted with chin-ups	3	8
Push-ups supersetted with pull-ups	3	8
Indian push-ups supersetted with body-weight shoulder presses	3	8
Plyometric jump squats supersetted with lunges	3	8
Single leg squats supersetted with free squats	3	8
Standing calf raises supersetted with hanging leg raises	3	8

bicycle ride or outside jog: 30 minutes

Note: The entire workout should be completed in 60 minutes or less.

Two Days a Week
Day 1, day 2: Full body, cardio

	Sets	Repetitions
Chin-ups supersetted with dips	3	8
Pull-ups supersetted with push-ups	3	8
Indian push-ups supersetted with body-weight shoulder presses	3	8

Plyometric jump squats supersetted with free squats	3	8
Lunges supersetted with single leg squats	3	8
Standing calf raises supersetted with leg raises	3	8

Outside jog or bicycle ride: 30 minutes

Note: The entire workout should be completed in 60 minutes or less.

One Day a Week
Day 1: Full body, cardio

	Sets	Repetitions
Pull-ups supersetted with push-ups	4	12
Chin-ups supersetted with dips	4	12
Indian push-ups supersetted with body-weight shoulder presses	4	12
Free squats supersetted with lunges	4	12
Plyometric jump squats supersetted with single leg raises	4	12
Standing calf raises supersetted with single leg squats	4	20

Outside jog: 30 minutes

Note: The entire workout should be completed in 75 minutes or less.

Chapter 15
Putting It All Together

Every person has a different schedule and different preferences, but there is always a training and diet regimen that will fit you perfectly. That's why this book has so many different exercise routines designed to be fun and interesting for beginning, intermediate, and advanced athletes.

The daily and weekly schedules I give vary depending on how many days you have available for serious exercise. My fitness formula differs from those of others in that regard: I give you flexibility in your choice of exercises and your schedule. Most other fitness professionals follow one method. Even though their methods have been successful in getting people into great shape, following the same approach all the times lacks variety. When your training regimen lacks variety, you begin to lose the fun factor. The fitness program starts to feel like a chore instead of an adventure. Once the process of getting into shape is no longer enjoyable, you lose interest and often end up quitting your fitness efforts altogether. Keeping the regimen as fun as possible will greatly increase your success rate..By following a custom-made program, you'll experience not only much greater success but will feel much more comfortable and have a much easier time following the program. You'll get into fantastic shape as effortlessly as possible.

Getting into shape is a lifestyle change, not a short-term diet and exercise program. People prefer to hear the words "lose weight fast" rather than "long-term fitness program," because most of us are in search of instant gratification. Having an attractive body and fantastic health is a rarity only because of the discipline and commitment required in order to achieve them.

The Four Phases

Now that you have all of the components of the first four phases in place, you are almost ready to move on to the last phase. To give you a recap of the prior phases, they are:

Phase I: making the decision that you will achieve the body and health you've long desired.

Phase II: Sleep; receive adequate sleep every night.

Phase III: Nutrition; eating well-balanced meals.

Phase IV: Exercise; incorporating both resistance and cardiovascular training.

Before we move on to the fifth and final stage, let's briefly go over the previous stages.

Phase I is the first and most important step because during this phase we decide that we no longer want to continue living out of shape. We must be clear to ourselves that we will take the necessary steps needed in order to achieve an optimum physique and health. We understand that the process will be prolonged, hence our lifestyles will need to change and head in a direction of health and fitness. This phase creates the proper foundation for the next phases to come. Through pure determination, perseverance, and commitment, you will achieve success.

Phase II is the simplest of all phases because it involves having proper rest and sufficient sleep. In order for the body to repair and rejuvenate itself, it must have enough rest. During sleep, the body physically and mentally replenishes itself, enabling it to perform at its best. With a good night's sleep you will feel stronger and your mind will be sharper. Your memory, reflexes, and muscular performance will all be noticeably better. With the proper amount of rest the body and mind can perform at their highest levels.

Phase III involves feeding the body with a nutritionally sound and well-balanced diet. Food for the body is equivalent to fuel for a race car. For a race car to operate at its best, the best possible fuel is necessary. The same applies to the body. For it to perform at its optimum level, you must eat a well-balanced diet. In order to achieve maximum results, each meal must contain the right amounts of protein, carbohydrates, and fat. Once you are eating consistent, well-balanced meals you will notice the difference—all of a sudden you will feel much more energetic and agile.

Phase IV is dedicated to exercising the body with both resistance training and cardiovascular workout routines. During this phase, you will begin to feel stronger and look more toned. Your body will now begin to look and feel years younger. The body's appetite and metabolism will increase and its immune system will improve as well. Due to the consistent exercising, you will have more drive to become much more active throughout the day.

Before moving on to the fifth and final phase it is very important to fully understand all of the components of all phases because each and every one plays an important role in achieving your fitness goals. Remember that the overall goal is to have the most fun possible while getting into the best shape of your life!

Combining the Phases for Success

With the four previous phases that have already been covered, we must now put them all together in order for your body to achieve its maximum potential. To simplify this process, I will format a complete weekly schedule for you to follow. Once you begin to follow the program, you will be well on your way to improving both your health and body to levels that you never thought were possible before. Remember to always have fun and enjoy the entire process of getting into shape. The journey is just as enjoyable as the results! You are now on your way!

I've already listed many possible meal and exercise options to choose from. Man or woman, vegan or omnivore, daily exercise or just once or twice a week—you now have the tools to create your own custom fitness program. Your program will take into account your goals, tastes, and lifestyle. As soon as you've designed a program that works well for you, however, it's time to start thinking about changing. Incorporating variety through frequent changes to your program keeps things interesting and also gives you the maximum results. Variety, fun, and results are three words that are always included into my fitness programs!

Your Fitness Schedule

I find that my clients get the best results if they stick to a regular meal and exercise schedule. You don't have to be rigid about your schedule, but try to eat and work out at roughly the same times every day. That includes rest days. If you've reached the advance stage, you may choose to divide your resistance training and cardiovascular training times and do them at different times

A regular schedule helps you stick with the program. It also helps you stick with the diet, because you eat regularly and predictably and don't ever have big gaps in your meal schedule that leave you feeling ravenous.

Before your workout, have a meal or snack—this gives you energy for the exercise. After your workout, you may not feel very hungry. Exercise is a great way to suppress your appetite. Within a couple of hours of completing your workout, however, you will need to refuel with another meal or snack.

The best time of day to exercise is the time that you like to exercise. Some people prefer early morning workouts so that they feel energized for the rest of the day. Others prefer to exercise at other times that are convenient for them, such as lunchtime or on the way home from work. The one time I don't recommend for exercise is before you go to sleep. Exercise is energizing and may keep you from falling asleep.

The Importance of Consistency

Consistency is crucial to success. In your nutrition, for instance, consistently fueling your body will optimize its ability to burn fat and remain energized throughout the entire day. A well-balanced diet will also help protect you from diseases such as hypertension and type 2 diabetes. Drinking plenty of water throughout the day will keep you well hydrated as well as provide your face with a healthy glow. A consistent, well-balanced meal plan, along with adequate sleep, will provide the body with enormous energy, causing you to look years younger.

Consistent exercise is an important part of the entire quality-of-life improvement package. Through resistance and cardiovascular training, your body will both strengthen and become more toned. Your metabolism will increase to the level of athletes years younger. Now you have accomplished in a few months what you have desired your entire life. You will feel strong, lean, toned, and filled with positive energy and enthusiasm. You are about to transcend into the fifth and final phase! Enjoy the journey because it may only come once in a lifetime!

Remember where you have started and where you are right now. When you look back, you will be amazed how much you have learned and how much you have changed and improved. The process and commitment aren't easy, but the results are well worth it. You have not only improved your health and body, you have also placed yourself into an entirely unique and elite category. You've become a person others both envy and admire. You will feel unique, young, and physically and mentally at a much higher level! The work has definitely paid off!

Chapter 16
Reaping The Benefits

Up until this point you have successfully transformed and improved your health and body. You've completed these phases:
Phase I: Making the choice (the mind)
Phase II: Sleep
Phase III: Nutrition
Phase IV: Exercise

This entire improvement process began with the first phase, which was deciding that you wanted to make this life-improving decision. You were living a life that was not 100 percent fulfilling and you wanted to finally take action to change. You realized that you weren't getting any younger. You now wanted to enjoy the best possible life and take full advantage of the years that remain. We all come to a point in our lives where we realize that life is shorter than what we had anticipated. We want to make the most of it.   To really maximize our lives, we must be willing to make major changes, beginning with lifestyle. These changes include diet, lifestyle, and exercise. We must be willing to make plenty of sacrifices and live in a more disciplined manner. We must commit 100 percent in order to reap the benefits of the quality of life that we are looking to live. During this phase, we accept we will commit 100 percent to a life of health and fitness in order to achieve our ultimate goal: improved quality of life!

During phase II, we prepare our bodies for an improved lifestyle, which begins by sleeping seven to eight hour a night. Having a sufficient amount of sleep enables your body to perform at the highest level, both physically and mentally. Your body will heal quickly from your workouts. Your mind will be relaxed, your mood will be enhanced, and your reflexes will be sharp.

Phase V

Congratulations! You have now graduated into the physically and mentally elite. All of your sacrifices and hard work have brought you to this point. It is now time to reap the rewards. The list of the rewards received from your hard work, commitment, and sacrifices is quite extensive. Most people only think of a few, such as the weight they lost or the stronger they feel. The truth is, a fitness program benefits you in so many more ways. The benefits extend to both the physical and the psychological: self-esteem and memory are improved, illnesses and diseases such as type w diabetes, osteoporosis, Alzheimer's disease, and many others may be slowed or prevented.

On the outside, you now look better: thinner, more muscular, more toned. You move more quickly, with more confidence and ease. But let's look at the internal physical improvements as well:

Stronger bones and joints
Stronger tendons and ligaments
Stronger heart; reduction in overall heart rate
Stronger arteries
Stronger lungs
Higher level of HDL "good" cholesterol
Lower level of triglycerides
Lower level of LDL (low density lipoprotein) cholesterol
Lower level of VLDL (very low density lipoprotein) cholesterol
Lower glucose level (blood sugar)
Increased antioxidant levels to help minimize free-radical damage
Increased cell and hormone efficiency
Faster reflexes
Less need for naps and excessive sleep
Increased metabolism
Faster healing from injuries and illnesses

Improved skin tone and elasticity
Increased overall energy
Improved blood circulation
Improved sexual function

Psychological Benefits

There are many psychological benefits to following a properly designed fitness plan. During exercise, the brain releases natural endorphins that make you feel extremely good. This is known as the exercise high or runner's high. This nice feeling begins to take effect within thirty minutes of exercising. It is what you should strive to achieve during each workout session. This high can sometimes last up to a full day, giving you a high level of energy and enthusiasm for everything you do.

Most people who follow a fitness regimen make the mistake of only concentrating on the physical changes of their bodies, rather than the psychological changes. You can immediately feel the exercise high, maybe even the very first time you do a real workout. The physical changes take longer to be noticeable. It will be a few weeks, for instance, before you notice that it is much easier to carry grocery bags into the house. It will probably be few months before you start to see real definition in your muscles.

You'll notice the psychological effects at once, however, both from the endorphins and from the improved energy and sense of self-worth you'll feel from day one. If you exercise every day, you experience positive results every day as well! The psychological benefits can be immediate and long-lasting, thus making your fitness program as fun and effortless as possible!

Phase V Benefits

The physical and psychological benefits that you will receive by following a well-designed meal plan are endless. During this final phase you are now beginning to reap the benefits of all your hard work and commitment. There is no doubt that this has been a long and well-fought journey, and now that you have accomplished your goal of being in phenomenal shape, having a well-toned and attractive body, great health, and a much happier state of mind, you are truly ready to live a much more fulfilling life.

Think back to where this journey began, when making the decision that you were going to get into the best shape of your life and that you would take every necessary step to do so and you would not be denied! Fast-forward to where you are today and you will look at yourself with pride and a sense of accomplishment! And you have absolutely every reason to do so! Looking back, it seemed rather easy, but starting all over again and looking ahead would seem as if it was a lifetime away!

The "new you" will feel completely different. You will feel better in every way possible, because you will look and feel much better both physically and mentally. Once in shape, other people will treat you different as well mainly because of a deep respect they will have for you, knowing how hard you worked to get to this point. Shopping for clothing will feel much better. You'll be looking at clothes that are a size or two smaller; you'll be able to wear clothes that make you look more attractive, increasing your overall mood. Everywhere you go, you will have more of a swagger to your walk—women feel this way, too. You will carry yourself in a manner that exudes confidence. Going to family get-togethers will be a lot more fun. You'll have more energy to have fun, joke around, and play with the kids.

Being in shape adds much more energy to your life. Going on vacations will be more fulfilling because you will need less nap time. Your body will feel more energized all day. You'll have more energy to sightsee, do physical things like kayaking and swimming, and still have energy in the evening to enjoy a nice dinner and some nightlife. Get ready to have more spark throughout your day!

You will notice many other quality of life improvements as well. Your posture, for instance, will improve. You will begin to notice that you stand up straighter and taller. Exercise improves posture and also adds confidence . You will walk, sit, speak to people, and carry yourself in a more confident and professional manner.

Confidence will also bring a new and positive attitude into your life. Words such as "I can't" will change to "I can and I will." Your outlook on life will change for the better. Now, you will look at a glass and see it as half full instead of half empty. Having a more positive attitude will drastically improve your quality of life. You will want to surround yourself with others who are positive as well. Your tolerance for associating with negative people will diminish, because you will realize how detrimental they are to your progress and physical and mental well-being. Maintaining a positive life could lead you to start new hobbies, do volunteer work, and be more active with your religious and community organizations. You might even decide to go back to school—you are never too old to learn. Check out your local community college and also courses and book groups through your local library, YMCA, and other organizations. You will keep you mind engaged while you expand your network of positive people and influences.

Set goals, work toward them, and never give up. If you have willpower, any dream is possible! Enjoy having the will to win, the will to be young at heart, and the will to thrive rather than just survive! When I was in college on the wrestling team, our practice room had many motivating slogans written along the padded walls. My favorite is one I think of every day: Believe and You Shall Achieve!

Enjoy the results of your hard work and accomplishments! From here on, each day will keep getting better. Maintaining your healthy lifestyle will become easier all the time. Continue to work hard and stay committed, and the physical and mental rewards you receive will continue as well. You only live once. Life is short, and youth is even shorter, so why not stay young for as long as you want? Because it truly is up to you!!

Go out there, turn back the clock, and have a beautiful and fulfilling life!! You earned it!